Table of Contents

Practice Test #1

Practice Questions

1. A patient has contracted chlamydia through unprotected sex. Which of the following is the most appropriate response?
   a. "It is a bacterial infection and can be treated with antibiotics."
   b. "You should abstain from sex until marriage."
   c. "There is no treatment for this disease."
   d. "Do not let anyone know you have this; it can ruin your reputation."

2. A patient with an external ventricular drain (EVD) has an intracranial pressure (ICP) of 30. The output of the drain is very sluggish when it is opened. What is the next step?
   a. Flush the drain proximally.
   b. Continue to monitor the ICP.
   c. Flush the drain distally.
   d. Call the attending/resident/PA.

3. While turning an 81-year-old nursing home patient, the nurse notices that the patient has a stage II decubitus ulcer on the right buttock. Which of the following is NOT a measure that the nurse should take in the treatment of the decubitus ulcer?
   a. Use of air mattresses
   b. Use of restraints
   c. Frequent turning
   d. Use of wet-to-dry dressings

4. Which of the following is recommended to help prevent the reoccurrence of kidney stones?
   a. Broccoli
   b. Steak
   c. Lemons
   d. Beer

5. A patient has just returned from the operating room. On the pre-operative orders the patient was ordered to receive Lopressor 25 mg po bid. On the post-operative orders the attending physician wrote for Lopressor 25 mg IV bid. The patient is due for the Lopressor dose. What is the next step in the nurse's management?
   a. Do not give Lopressor.
   b. Give the po dose.
   c. Give the IV dose.
   d. Call the attending to clarify the order.

6. Which of the following is NOT a risk factor for developing a decubitus ulcer?
   a. Bowel or bladder retention
   b. Diabetes mellitus
   c. Aging skin
   d. Peripheral vascular disease

7. A nurse has just placed a nasogastric tube in a patient. Which of the following would be expected to be ordered after nasogastric tube placement?
   a. Abdominal ultrasound
   b. Chest x-ray
   c. Abdominal x-ray
   d. EKG

8. Which of the following treatments is the most important when treating a patient who is hypotensive and lethargic?
   a. Obtaining a CT scan of the brain
   b. Obtaining a pan culture
   c. Maintaining the airway
   d. Administering a fluid bolus

9. A woman calls the unit and identifies herself as a patient's cousin and asks how the patient fared overnight. The patient is unable to communicate. The patient's power of attorney and only known family member is her husband. What should be your response?
   a. Give her a brief synopsis of how the patient is doing.
   b. Apologize, but explain to the cousin that you cannot give out the information.
   c. Give the cousin your patient's husband's phone number and instruct her to speak to him.
   d. Give her directions to the hospital and request that she speak to you in person since you cannot give that information over the phone.

10. You are caring for a patient who ruptured his spleen in a motor vehicle accident and required a splenectomy. Identify the vaccine you expect to administer after surgery:
   a. Recombivax HB
   b. Attenuvax
   c. Pneumovax 23
   d. Tetanus toxoid

11. A patient is scheduled for an evacuation of a small subdural hematoma the following morning. He is scheduled to receive a Lantus dose at 11 pm and was ordered to be NPO past midnight. What is the next step in your management?
   a. Give the Lantus.
   b. Give half the dose of Lantus.
   c. Hold the Lantus.
   d. Call the attending to clarify the order.

12. What are the four most fundamental needs or deficiency needs according to Maslow's hierarchy?
   a. Sleep, exercise, healthy weight, nutritious diet
   b. Food, water, sleep, excretion
   c. Money, sex, love, sleep
   d. Money, water, love, exercise

13. Which of the following is NOT a common reason for post-operative fever that occurs within one week of surgery?
    a. Line infection
    b. Urinary tract infection
    c. Wound infection
    d. Deep vein thrombosis

14. After a patient's death, the family is grieving. The patient's mother states that she is overwhelmed and doesn't know how to proceed since she has never had a death in the family before. Which of the following would NOT be a suggestion you would make to the patient's family member?
    a. Call the family's religious leader for support.
    b. Recommend grief counseling groups.
    c. Recommend starting anti-depressant medications.
    d. Call the hospital social worker.

15. Which of the following is the most common cause of ketoacidosis?
    a. Hyperglycemia
    b. Hypertension
    c. Hypoxia
    d. Dehydration

16. All of the following are true about sickle cell anemia EXCEPT:
    a. It is a genetic disease.
    b. It increases risk for stroke and heart attack.
    c. It can be diagnosed with a complete blood count (CBC).
    d. Treatment includes blood transfusion and oxygen.

17. What is the most common side effect seen with the use of clopidogrel?
    a. Cough
    b. Hypotension
    c. Erectile dysfunction
    d. Bleeding

18. Your patient is admitted with a history of peptic ulcer disease and vomiting for several days. His arterial blood gas (ABG) results are: pH 7.52; $PaCO_2$ 49 mm/Hg; PaO_2 62 mm/ Hg; and HCO_3^- 40 mEq/L. He has a nasogastric tube inserted. Identify the condition your patient is experiencing:
    a. Metabolic acidosis
    b. Metabolic alkalosis
    c. Respiratory acidosis
    d. Respiratory alkalosis

19. In response to being told that she has terminal lung cancer, a patient states "Well I really don't feel that sick; you must be mistaken regarding my diagnosis." Which stage of Kübler-Ross's five stages of grief would best describe this patient?
    a. Anger
    b. Denial
    c. Bargaining
    d. Acceptance

20. What is the most important recommendation that can be given to a patient prior to receiving the bowel prep for a colonoscopy?
    a. Stop taking your medications prior to the procedure.
    b. Eat a pureed diet only during the prep.
    c. Eat red foods/fluids.
    d. It is important to remain hydrated.

21. All of the following are recommendations to prevent an asthma attack EXCEPT:
    a. "Keep away from pet dander."
    b. "Treat upper respiratory infections quickly."
    c. "If you smoke, smoke outside the house."
    d. "Avoid strong fragrances."

22. What is NOT a common side effect seen with the long-term use of prednisone?
    a. Skin atrophy
    b. Impaired immune response
    c. Diabetes
    d. Orange urine

23. Identify the electrolyte imbalance most likely to affect a patient with Crohn's disease:
    a. Hyperkalemia
    b. Hypermagnesemia
    c. Hypokalemia
    d. Hypomagnesemia

24. Your patient is a chronic alcoholic with hypomagnesemia. Select another electrolyte imbalance that may result from a magnesium deficiency:
    a. Hypercalcemia
    b. Hypernatremia
    c. Hypokalemia
    d. Hypophosphatemia

25. A nurse is treating a patient with *C. difficile* colitis. Which of the following are the most important measures to prevent the spread of the disease to herself/himself and other patients?
    a. Goggles and gown
    b. Gloves and gown
    c. Hand washing and gloves
    d. Face mask and gloves

26. Which of the following foods should be avoided to help to prevent listeriosis?
    a. Chocolate
    b. Pasteurized milk
    c. Soda
    d. Hot dogs

27. You administer nalbuphine hydrochloride (Nubain), an opiate antagonist, to your patient for pain control. Choose the sign(s) that triggers you to further assess your patient for opiate dependence:
    a. Respiratory depression
    b. Nausea and vomiting
    c. Gooseflesh and diarrhea
    d. Seizures

28. Which of the following is the best method to treat scabies?
    a. Application of permethrin
    b. Application of Lamisil
    c. Condoms
    d. Hand washing

29. Which of the following is the least likely to cause a cardiac arrest?
    a. Trauma
    b. Trichomoniasis
    c. Toxins
    d. Tamponade

30. During which phase of the nursing process does a nurse prioritize addressing a patient's medical issues according to their severity?
    a. Diagnosing
    b. Planning
    c. Implementing
    d. Evaluating

31. What is the primary treatment of cystic fibrosis?
    a. Chemotherapy and radiation
    b. Maintain ideal body mass index
    c. Symptomatic relief
    d. Surgical intervention

32. In response to being told that she has terminal lung cancer, the patient states "If I stop smoking I think you will be able to cure me." Which stage of Kübler-Ross's five stages of grief would best describe this patient?
    a. Depression
    b. Acceptance
    c. Anger
    d. Bargaining

33. Among the following signs and symptoms, which would be the least likely to be present in a patient with acute asthma exacerbation?
    a. Low-grade fever
    b. Chest pain
    c. Shortness of breath
    d. Tinnitus

34. A patient suddenly develops diffuse extremity tremors, drooling, eye-rolling, and does not respond to verbal or tactile stimuli for several minutes. The episode resolves spontaneously and afterward the patient is confused and lethargic. What type of seizure did this patient most likely experience?
    a. Petit mal seizure
    b. Tonic-clonic seizure
    c. Absence seizure
    d. Simple partial seizure

35. A patient with multiple lower-extremity fractures following a motorcycle crash has a cast placed on the affected extremity. Which of the following is the most serious complication that could result from this patient's injury?
    a. Compartment syndrome
    b. Deep vein thrombosis
    c. Muscle weakness
    d. Arthritis

36. A nurse is caring for a patient with a potential acute cerebral vascular accident. The symptoms started two hours ago. The CT scan of the head shows a hemorrhagic infarct. Which of the following should the nurse expect to be the next step in the physician's management?
    a. Order aspirin and Plavix.
    b. Repeat a CT scan in the morning.
    c. Administer tissue plasminogen activator (tPA).
    d. Discharge the patient home.

37. What is primary cause of a celiac sprue exacerbation?
    a. Alcohol
    b. Green leafy vegetables
    c. Dehydration
    d. Gluten-based products

38. Which of the following plays an important role in confirming the diagnosis of septic arthritis?
    a. X-ray
    b. 2D echo
    c. Blood cultures
    d. NSAIDs

39. Which of the following is the highest-level need according to Maslow's hierarchy?
    a. Sexual intimacy
    b. Self-actualization
    c. Security
    d. Sleep

40. Which of the following foods would NOT be recommended in a patient with a history of fecal impaction?
    a. Raspberries
    b. Fish
    c. Lentils
    d. Oatmeal

41. Your patient's diagnosis is hypernatremia. The primary treatment for this patient is:
    a. Sodium polystyrene sulfonate (Kayexalate)
    b. Fluid replacement
    c. Diuretics
    d. Activated charcoal

42. Following an open appendectomy a patient is unable to pass a bowel movement and has persistent nausea and vomiting. Which of the following should the nurse suspect as the most likely diagnosis?
    a. Ileus
    b. Intussusception
    c. Toxic megacolon
    d. *C. difficile* colitis

43. A patient recently diagnosed with gout asks his nurse about what he can do to reduce the prevalence of gout attacks. Which of the following dietary recommendations should the nurse NOT recommend?
    a. Reduce coffee intake.
    b. Increase seafood intake.
    c. Reduce calcium intake.
    d. Increase fructose intake.

44. A patient in the hospital for a subdural hematoma was previously able to follow commands and is now only localizing to pain. The patient's next dose of Percocet is due now. Which of the following should be the first step in intervention?
    a. Order a CT scan of the brain.
    b. Reassess exam in 30 minutes.
    c. Give the patient the Percocet.
    d. Call the attending.

45. A patient is being discharged on Coumadin. Which of the following foods should the nurse recommend that the patient limit?
    a. Fructose
    b. Kale
    c. Yogurt
    d. Gluten-based products

46. Which of the following interventions would NOT help prevent acute sickle cell crisis?
    a. Limit alcohol use.
    b. Avoid cigarette smoke.
    c. Exercise regularly.
    d. Exposure to cold.

47. A patient recovering from an acute myocardial infarction asks his nurse why he was given aspirin. What is the most appropriate response?
    a. "It decreases workload on the heart."
    b. "It causes vasodilation."
    c. "It prevents clot formation."
    d. "It thins out the blood."

48. A 30-year-old patient is being seen in the ER today for a wrist fracture. His blood pressure is 138/88. He smokes half a pack of cigarettes per day. His other vital signs are normal. Which of the following is the most appropriate intervention?
    a. Monitor for now; recommend limiting tobacco.
    b. Recommend an electrocardiogram.
    c. Recommend use of antihypertensive medications.
    d. Recommend use of an inhaler.

49. A patient presents to the hospital with suspected pneumothorax. Which of the following tests would confirm the diagnosis?
    a. Electrocardiogram
    b. Echocardiogram
    c. Chest x-ray
    d. Blood cultures

50. A patient who was admitted for an acute exacerbation of congestive heart failure asks why she is being discharged on Lasix. What is the most appropriate response?
    a. "It prevents excessive edema."
    b. "It increases vasodilation."
    c. "It prevents clots."
    d. "It reduces inflammation."

51. Patients being discharged on Lasix should increase their intake of which of the following foods?
    a. Corn
    b. Watermelon
    c. Carrots
    d. Bananas

52. A patient notes that he has a family history of diabetes. His fasting blood sugar is 138 and his HbA1c is 6.2. What should the nurse expect the attending to recommend for this patient?
    a. Recheck his HbA1c in a week.
    b. Recommend low sugar diet and exercise.
    c. Start Lantus and metformin.
    d. Start levothyroxine.

53. A 45-year-old female with no remarkable past medical history has never had a colonoscopy. When should the nurse advise this patient to get her first colonoscopy?
    a. This year
    b. At age 70
    c. At age 60
    d. At age 50

54. A patient is suspected to have a pulmonary embolism. Which of the following tests should the nurse NOT expect to be ordered?
    a. Echocardiogram
    b. Chest x-ray
    c. Arterial blood gas
    d. Ventilation perfusion scan

55. Your patient sustained a fracture of the left femur in a motorcycle accident and developed a fat embolism. Select the laboratory findings you expect:
    a. Decreased serum lipase levels
    b. Decreased erythrocyte sedimentation rate
    c. Decreased red blood cell and platelet counts
    d. Increased serum albumin and calcium levels

56. A few minutes after you change a patient's total parenteral nutrition (TPN) tubing, he complains of chest pain and shortness of breath. His pulse is weak and thready. Identify the top priority intervention:
    a. Turn the patient on his left side, with his head lower than his body
    b. Call a Code Blue and initiate cardiopulmonary resuscitation (CPR)
    c. Stop the TPN and keep the line open with saline solution
    d. Notify the physician because the patient is having an allergic reaction

57. Your diabetic patient is hypertensive. Treatment is carvedilol (Coreg). Select the instruction to emphasize to your patient during discharge teaching:
    a. Check pulses daily because carvedilol causes tachycardia
    b. Resume vigorous foot care because carvedilol decreases perfusion
    c. Monitor blood sugar levels because carvedilol masks signs of hypoglycemia
    d. Monitor blood sugar levels because carvedilol may cause hyperglycemia

58. Three days after surgery, your patient develops a low-grade fever and a tender, swollen calf. Choose the most appropriate intervention:
    a. Tell the physician
    b. Massage the calf
    c. Ambulate the patient
    d. Perform range of motion (ROM) exercises on the legs

59. Which of the following is a common risk factor for developing condyloma acuminata?
    a. Family history
    b. IV drug abuse
    c. Smoking
    d. Multiple pregnancies

60. A patient has a deficiency of human growth hormone. Which of the following will be the most likely diagnosis?
    a. Gigantism
    b. Dwarfism
    c. Diabetes
    d. Acromegaly

61. A patient is admitted to the hospital for multiple extremity and rib fractures after a fall that occurred today. A CT scan of the head is negative. He has a known history of alcohol abuse. He is oriented to person and place but not the year. His speech is slurred. His alcohol level is 396. He denies drug abuse. Based on his history and physical exam, what is the most likely diagnosis?

    a. Delusional disorder
    b. Alcohol intoxication
    c. Alcohol withdrawal
    d. Depression

62. A patient being discharged on Pyridium should be advised of which of the following side effects?

    a. Bright orange urine
    b. Bleeding
    c. Tinnitus
    d. Angioedema

63. A newborn is diagnosed with phenylketonuria (PKU). Which of the following should be avoided?

    a. Protein
    b. Fruit
    c. Juices
    d. Vegetables

64. Which of the following patients should NOT get the flu vaccine?

    a. A 46-year-old man who smokes half a pack per day
    b. A 2-month-old child
    c. A 33-year-old pregnant patient
    d. An 89-year-old patient with no significant past medical history

65. Your patient is hospitalized for a stroke and experiences homonymous hemianopsia on her left side. Choose the most important intervention:

    a. Approach the patient on her left side
    b. Speak clearly into the patient's right ear
    c. Teach the patient to scan her visual field
    d. Have the patient chew slowly and thoroughly before swallowing

66. A pediatric patient has just been diagnosed with thalassemia major. Which of the following is a common complication?

    a. Obesity
    b. Diabetes
    c. Heart failure
    d. Cataracts

67. A patient is diagnosed with moderate iron deficiency anemia. Aside from iron supplements, of which of the following should the patient increase her intake?

    a. Yogurt
    b. Pasta
    c. Oranges
    d. Broccoli

68. A patient with hypovolemic shock should be placed in which of the following positions to help increase blood pressure?
   a. Prone
   b. Lithotomy
   c. Supine
   d. Trendelenburg

69. A patient is suspected of having compartment syndrome. Which of the following tests should the nurse expect to be initially ordered?
   a. CT scan
   b. Arterial Doppler
   c. MRI
   d. X-ray

70. A patient who arrived at the hospital as a trauma alert and initially was an 11 on the Glasgow Coma Scale (GCS) undergoes a neurological change and now has a GCS of 3. The telemetry monitor shows that the patient is in pulseless ventricular tachycardia. What should be the first step in taking care of this patient?
   a. Intubate the patient.
   b. Get a CT scan of the brain.
   c. Administer atropine.
   d. Administer epinephrine.

71. A nurse suspects that her patient's chest tube unit has an air leak. Which of the following interventions would be appropriate?
   a. Pull out the tube.
   b. Administer Dermabond around the incision site.
   c. Use rubber-tipped clamps to momentarily clamp the tubing.
   d. Strip or "milk" the tubing.

72. A nurse is taking care of a patient with a traumatic brain injury. The patient has developed a steadily increasing intracranial pressure. Which of the following medications should the nurse expect to be given to this patient?
   a. Lantus
   b. Levothyroxine
   c. Lanoxin
   d. Lasix

73. Your patient is hospitalized with a possible diagnosis of Guillain-Barré syndrome. Indicate the question you should ask when collecting history data from your patient:
   a. "Do you bruise easily?"
   b. "Have you had an upper respiratory tract infection recently?"
   c. "Have you been out of the country during the past 4 months?"
   d. "Has anyone in your family ever had Guillain-Barré syndrome?"

74. A male patient is brought to the hospital with sudden-onset unilateral testicular pain following a trauma that occurred four hours ago. What diagnosis should the nurse suspect?
    a. Testicular carcinoma
    b. Testicular torsion
    c. Varicocele
    d. Hydrocele

75. A patient suddenly loses consciousness and is found to be in pulseless ventricular tachycardia. All of the following medications may be administered EXCEPT
    a. magnesium sulfate.
    b. lidocaine.
    c. dopamine.
    d. amiodarone.

76. A patient admitted for a stroke is due for his dose of a full aspirin. The patient has failed his swallow evaluation. What should the nurse do?
    a. Cancel the aspirin order.
    b. Crush the aspirin and give it to him with applesauce.
    c. Skip the dose.
    d. Get an order to give it to the patient per rectum.

77. A patient admitted for stroke has failed his swallow evaluation for two consecutive days. Which of the following should the nurse suggest to the medical team in regards to the patient's nutrition?
    a. Pureed diet
    b. Liquid diet
    c. Tube feeds
    d. Total parenteral nutrition

78. A 25-year-old female is admitted to the hospital for attempted suicide. She admits to rapid mood swings alternating between feelings of euphoria and severe depression. What is the most likely diagnosis?
    a. Anorexia nervosa
    b. Bulimia nervosa
    c. Generalized anxiety disorder
    d. Bipolar disorder

79. A patient who has just undergone a lumbar puncture is now complaining of headache and dizziness. Which of the positions would help alleviate the symptoms?
    a. Supine
    b. Fowler's
    c. Reverse Trendelenburg
    d. Sitting

80. Which of the following medications should the nurse give to a patient with supraventricular tachycardia according to ACLS protocol?
    a. Norvasc
    b. Tylenol
    c. Morphine
    d. Adenosine

81. The NANDA-I classification system is used to organize which of the following?
    a. Diagnoses
    b. Assessments
    c. Plans
    d. Interventions

82. A patient is admitted to the unit after a traumatic brain injury. The nurse notices that the patient has developed foot drop. Which of the following is the most appropriate intervention?
    a. Daily massage of the affected extremity
    b. Placement of an orthopedic boot
    c. Elevation of the foot on a pillow
    d. Placement of an elastic stocking

83. A patient with osteopenia asks her nurse how to prevent progression of the disease. Which of the following is the best advice the nurse can give to this patient?
    a. Increasing fluid intake
    b. Wearing thick layers of clothing
    c. Limiting intake of red meat and alcohol
    d. Increasing calcium intake

84. A nurse notices that a patient has pain while the doctor palpates the patient's left costovertebral angle. Which of the following is the most likely diagnosis?
    a. Small bowel obstruction
    b. Appendicitis
    c. Pyelonephritis
    d. Cholecystitis

85. What does Reynold's pentad include?
    a. Wheezing, nonproductive cough, fever, chest pain, hypoxia
    b. RUQ pain, fever, jaundice, hypotension, and confusion
    c. Back pain, fever, chills, anorexia, and vomiting
    d. Dysuria, hematuria, penile discharge, fever, skin lesions

86. A patient with cystic fibrosis asks her nurse what medications she can take for symptomatic relief. Which of the following medications should the nurse NOT advise this patient to use?
    a. Motrin
    b. Permethrin
    c. Colace
    d. Emollients

87. A patient confides in his nurse that he wants to commit suicide. He tells the nurse how and when he plans to do it. Which of the following is NOT an appropriate action as a medical professional?
    a. Advise the patient to call a suicide hotline.
    b. Obtain a stat psychiatric referral.
    c. Do not report the patient's actions.
    d. Advise the patient's spouse or parents of his intent.

88. A 22-year-old patient is being discharged from the hospital with a long leg cast due to a broken femur. Which of the following should NOT occur three months after hospital discharge?
    a. Performing self-care activities independently
    b. Ambulating independently
    c. Participating in physical therapy
    d. Riding a motorcycle

89. A patient is admitted to the hospital for cardiac arrhythmias and muscle weakness. An EKG shows peaked T waves. The patient has a known history of chronic renal insufficiency and has been taking an angiotensin converting enzyme (ACE) inhibitor for his high blood pressure. Which of the following best describes what the patient's electrolytes may look like?
    a. K 5.6, creatinine 1.4, BUN 28
    b. BUN 35, K 4.9, creatinine 2.3
    c. K 6.5, creatinine 1.0, BUN 16
    d. Creatinine 0.9, K 3.1, BUN 7

90. A patient has been diagnosed with an upper extremity superficial vein thrombus. Which of the following would be a part of the medical management?
    a. Lovenox
    b. Compression stockings
    c. Coumadin
    d. Warm compresses

91. Which of the following is NOT a treatment of thalassemia major?
    a. Folate supplements
    b. Chelation therapy
    c. Blood transfusions
    d. Lumbar puncture

92. Which of the following is not a sign or symptom of Cushing's disease?
    a. Acromegaly
    b. Obesity
    c. Skin striae
    d. Facial edema

93. Which of the following treatments is NOT an intervention for a patient with acute alcohol intoxication?
    a. Zofran
    b. Folate
    c. Thiamine
    d. Ativan

94. An 88-year-old female develops left-sided weakness and is brought to the ER. She is diagnosed with a stroke and receives tissue plasminogen activator (tPA) in the ER and develops a hemorrhagic stroke. The patient is taken to the OR for an evacuation of the intracerebral hemorrhage and a small surgical instrument is accidentally left inside the patient's head. The patient develops a brain abscess and has to return to the OR for a second surgery. Which of the following is the sentinel event?
    a. The ischemic stroke
    b. The hemorrhagic stroke
    c. The surgical error
    d. The brain abscess

95. A patient is diagnosed with a pneumothorax. Which of the following would the nurse NOT expect to be an intervention for this patient?
    a. Warm compresses
    b. Supplemental oxygen
    c. Narcotics
    d. Chest tube

96. A patient is newly diagnosed with gastroesophageal reflux disease and prescribed esomeprazole. Which of the following is an accurate explanation of the drug's action?
    a. "It slows down digestion."
    b. "It prevents peristalsis."
    c. "It coats the stomach lining to prevent acid erosion."
    d. "It decreases the production of stomach acid."

97. A patient is admitted to the hospital with pelvic inflammatory disease. What is one of the most common complications of pelvic inflammatory disease?
    a. Appendicitis
    b. Multiple births
    c. Infertility
    d. Bleeding

98. Your patient is wearing a cervical collar after a motor vehicle accident. The radiologist has not checked his cervical x-ray results yet. Which bed position is best for your patient?
    a. Flat
    b. High Fowler's
    c. Trendelenburg
    d. Reverse Trendelenburg

99. Which of the following will not help alleviate the symptoms of premenstrual syndrome?
    a. Exercise
    b. Dietary modifications
    c. Birth control pills
    d. Caffeine

100. Which of the following may help prevent cervical cancer?
    a. Routine testing for venereal disease
    b. Refraining from using diaphragms
    c. Avoiding alcohol
    d. Limiting the number of sexual partners

101. Which of the following is NOT a complication of beriberi?
    a. Muscle weakness
    b. Diabetes
    c. Encephalopathy
    d. Seizures

102. Which of the following is the best way to prevent diabetes mellitus?
    a. Decrease processed foods.
    b. Increase thiamine intake.
    c. Decrease alcohol intake.
    d. Increase iron intake.

103. A 48 year old awake and alert patient on your unit normally manages his diabetes with Novolin R sliding scale insulin. His wife is helping him get his lunch tray set up when the nurse assistant reports to you that his blood sugar is 68. He did not receive any insulin. Which of the following would be the least appropriate intervention for this patient?
    a. Administer D5W.
    b. Encourage intake of lunch, especially long and short acting carbohydrates.
    c. Recheck blood sugar in 30 minutes.
    d. Advise the patient to avoid rising quickly or walking until after his blood sugar has stabilized, and his wife to report and change in mental status.

104. A patient who has suffered a stroke is being discharged home today. The patient's wife is concerned about caring for her husband at home. Which of the following is NOT an appropriate response to the patient's wife?
    a. "He should gradually increase his activity as tolerated."
    b. "I can help coordinate referrals for various medical specialists."
    c. "He should be on bed rest except for bathing or toileting."
    d. "If there is any change in his neurological status please call 911."

105. A patient develops a fever and mild chest pain and develops a generalized body rash while being transfused with blood. Which of the following should be the nurse's first step in this patient's management?
    a. Administer Benadryl.
    b. Stop the transfusion.
    c. Administer Tylenol.
    d. Perform an EKG.

106. A patient is admitted to the hospital for a pulmonary embolus likely caused by her sickle cell disease. She is placed on a heparin infusion and started on Coumadin. While on anticoagulation the patient develops massive epistaxis requiring a blood transfusion. The patient develops a hemolytic transfusion reaction because she was transfused with the wrong blood type. Which of the following is the sentinel event?
    a. Sickle cell disease
    b. Pulmonary embolus
    c. Epistaxis
    d. Transfusion

107. A patient with a subarachnoid hemorrhage has developed vasospasm. Which of the following would help prevent further complication?
    a. Maintaining elevated blood pressure
    b. Applying warm compresses
    c. Administering antihypertensive medication
    d. Maintaining euvolemia

108. Which of the following is the most appropriate intervention for an ileus?
    a. Trickle feeds
    b. Surgery
    c. Narcotic pain medications
    d. Transfusions

109. Which of the following is NOT a phase in the nurse-client therapeutic relationship?
    a. Uncooperative stage
    b. Orientation stage
    c. Exploration stage
    d. Termination stage

110. A patient is being treated with Pradaxa. Which of the following is one of the most common dangerous side effects?
    a. Liver failure
    b. Bleeding
    c. Ototoxicity
    d. Cough

111. Which of the following does OBRA regulate?
    a. Medical malpractice limits
    b. The care of nursing home residents
    c. Herbal medicine
    d. Medical waste laws

112. Which of the following two medications should NOT be taken together?
    a. Lopressor and Norvasc
    b. Metformin and Lantus
    c. Aspirin and Lasix
    d. Nexium and Plavix

113. A patient with Sjögren's syndrome asks her nurse which medications she can take to help decrease the severity of her symptoms. Which of the following should the nurse suggest?
    a. NSAIDs and birth control pills
    b. Albuterol and Atrovent
    c. Saline nasal spray and eye drops
    d. Benadryl and Decadron

114. A nurse is taking care of a patient with bilateral lower extremity superficial vein thromboses (SVTs). Which of the following should NOT be ordered for this patient?
    a. Repeat lower extremity ultrasound Dopplers
    b. Subcutaneous heparin or Lovenox
    c. Bed rest
    d. Placement of an inferior vena cava filter (IVCF)

115. Which of the following interventions would NOT help treat a patient in status epilepticus?
    a. Finger sweep the mouth for obstruction
    b. Reverse Trendelenburg
    c. Supplemental oxygen
    d. Antiepileptic medications

116. A nurse is caring for a patient with a known history of anxiety. She is scheduled for an MRI later that day and the patient tearfully tells the nurse that she is very claustrophobic. Which of the following medications should the nurse ask to be ordered for the patient prior to undergoing the test?
    a. Lorazepam
    b. Lantus
    c. Levoxyl
    d. Lopressor

117. Which of the following medications would be used for a person diagnosed with bipolar disorder?
    a. Decadron
    b. Lantus
    c. Permethrin
    d. Lexapro

118. A patient with advanced cirrhosis is admitted with bleeding esophageal varices and associated hepatic encephalopathy. You expect to give neomycin to:
    a. Control secondary infection in the hepatic bile ducts
    b. Prevent the development of bacterial bronchitis and pneumonia
    c. Eliminate microorganisms from the kidney, ureters, and bladder
    d. Destroy intestinal organisms that break down proteins to ammonia

119. Which of the following scenarios would NOT require RhoGAM administration?
    a. A mother with AB- blood whose fetus is AB+
    b. A fetus with O+ blood whose mother is A-
    c. A mother with B- blood whose fetus is O+
    d. A fetus with A- blood whose mother is B-

120. A surgical nurse accidentally sticks herself with a needle during surgery. The patient has a known history of hepatitis C. Which of the following actions is NOT advisable?
    a. Continue assisting with the surgery.
    b. Notify the patient of the incident once he/she is conscious.
    c. Notify Employee Health and a supervisor.
    d. Immediately scrub out of the procedure.

121. You are assessing your patient with a history of hepatitis. Choose how to evaluate her for asterixis:
    a. Instruct the patient to squat
    b. Measure the patient's abdominal girth
    c. Ask the patient to hyperextend her feet
    d. Ask the patient to extend her arm and hyperextend her hand

122. A patient begins to choke while she is eating her food. Her face starts turning bright red, but she is able to cough. Which of the following should be the next course of action?
    a. Start performing abdominal thrusts.
    b. Begin back slaps.
    c. Allow the patient to drink small sips of water.
    d. Perform finger sweeps of the mouth to remove the food.

123. A patient is in the process of being directly admitted to a unit from the doctor's office. The only orders on his chart so far are admit the patient to medical surgical unit, stat lab work, bedrest, and NPO status. The patient's daughters are at his side and he is talking to the registrar when he starts seizing. Which of the following is NOT an appropriate action by the nurse?
    a. Administer a Dilantin bolus.
    b. Place the patient on his side.
    c. Call the attending/admitting physician.
    d. Ask the family members to please step outside.

124. Your patient with a history of alcohol abuse is hospitalized with acute pancreatitis. Choose the finding you expect:
    a. Chvostek's sign
    b. Shortness of breath
    c. Hyperactive bowel sounds
    d. Decreased serum glucose level

125. Which of the following foods/drinks should a patient with frequent episodes of acid reflux avoid?
    a. Tea
    b. Oatmeal
    c. Fennel
    d. Wine

126. Your patient with gallbladder disease develops acute pancreatitis. What drug-free pain relief measure is appropriate for this patient?
    a. Encourage ambulation
    b. Give frequent, small sips of milk
    c. Place a heating pad over the epigastrium
    d. Have the patient lie in a lateral decubitus knee-bent position

127. Your patient with a history of Hepatitis C now has a total bilirubin level of 2.3 mg/dl, elevated liver enzyme levels, ascites, and jaundice. Nursing interventions for this patient should include:
    a. Frequent meals
    b. Daily mouth care
    c. Increased activity
    d. Frequent repositioning

128. Which of the following is the most appropriate test for measuring intraocular pressure?
    a. Calorimetry
    b. Fluorescein screen
    c. Spirometry
    d. Tonometry

129. Select the condition that may occur in your patient who is receiving total parenteral nutrition:
    a. Hypoglycemia
    b. Metabolic acidosis
    c. Metabolic alkalosis
    d. Hyperphosphatemia

130. A patient with a history of I.V. drug abuse and acute Hepatitis B now has with shallow, labored respirations, and severe ascites. Choose the intervention that best relieves respiratory distress caused by ascites:
    a. Nasopharyngeal suction
    b. Placing the patient in a supine position
    c. Administering diuretics, as prescribed, and maintaining sodium restriction
    d. Maintaining a low protein and fat-restricted diet

131. A patient is made Comfort Measures Only (CMO) by family members. Which of the following medications should be given to help control the patient's tachycardia?
    a. Amiodarone
    b. Morphine
    c. Lopressor
    d. Digoxin

132. A nurse coming on for the night shift is assigned to a patient who had an open cholecystectomy approximately 10 hours ago. The patient is awake, alert, and oriented. Which of the following complaints from the patient should be most concerning to the night nurse?
    a. "My appetite is not the same as it is normally."
    b. "I have a moderate amount of abdominal pain."
    c. "I haven't been able to urinate since I got out of surgery."
    d. "It hurts to cough or sneeze."

133. Choose the intervention that is most important to perform before a patient undergoes surgery to correct a complete small bowel obstruction:
   a. Ensure proper fluid and electrolyte replacement
   b. Teach the patient about ileostomy care
   c. Obtain informed consent for the procedure
   d. Begin total parenteral nutrition (TPN)

134. A patient receiving intravenous vancomycin develops erythema on her face, neck, hands, and feet. She also reports mild nausea. She denies pruritus, shortness of breath, or chest pain. Her vital signs are stable. She has no history of drug allergies. Which of the following is the most appropriate first step?
   a. Administer supplemental oxygen.
   b. Continue the infusion of vancomycin.
   c. Administer Benadryl.
   d. Discontinue the vancomycin.

135. A patient confides in his nurse that he may have AIDS, but he has never been checked. Which of the following tests would confirm the diagnosis?
   a. India ink
   b. Western blot
   c. Mantoux
   d. Rapid Plasma Reagin (RPR)

136. A patient with which of the following lab values would benefit from being prescribed a statin?
   a. LDL 165, HDL 65, Triglycerides 200
   b. HDL 55, Triglycerides 155, LDL 135
   c. HDL 60, LDL 120, Triglycerides 150
   d. Triglycerides 130, LDL 100, HDL 50

137. When caring for a patient with acute pancreatitis, you should be alert for:
   a. Hypercalcemia
   b. Acute respiratory distress syndrome (ARDS)
   c. Pericarditis
   d. Diabetes insipidus

138 A nurse is caring for a patient who is suspected to have diabetes mellitus. Which of the following tests would aid in the diagnosis?
   a. Thyroid function tests
   b. Complete blood count
   c. Cortisol level
   d. HbA1c

139. You are caring for a patient with hepatic failure due to liver cancer. The patient's prothrombin time is 56 seconds. You should expect to administer:
   a. Heparin
   b. Protamine sulfate
   c. Packed red blood cells
   d. Phytonadione (Vitamin K)

140. A patient who has Hashimoto's disease asks his nurse what the most common cause is for this condition. Which of the following is the most appropriate response?
 a. Autoimmune disorder
 b. Hormone imbalances
 c. Lack of physical exercise
 d. Cancer

141. A nurse is examining a patient with suspected osteomyelitis. Which of the following is the best test to help aid in the diagnosis?
 a. MRI
 b. Ultrasound
 c. X-ray
 d. EKG

142. A mother pregnant with her first child is Rh negative. The child is Rh negative. What is the next step in medical management?
 a. Antibiotics
 b. Transvaginal ultrasound
 c. No intervention
 d. RhoGAM

143. A patient is diagnosed with trichomoniasis. Which of the following is the most appropriate preventative therapy?
 a. Use birth control pills.
 b. Practice safe sex.
 c. Refrain from eating uncooked pork.
 d. Limit alcohol use.

144. A student is helping a nurse care for a patient with an intracerebral hemorrhage with moderate surrounding edema. He asks his preceptor if there are any IV fluids that would be contraindicated in this patient. Which of the following would be the most appropriate answer?
 a. D5W
 b. Lactated Ringer's
 c. Normal saline
 d. 3% NaCl

145. A 24-year-old patient newly diagnosed with uterine fibroids asks her nurse what therapies should alleviate her symptoms. Which of the following is NOT an appropriate response?
 a. NSAIDs
 b. Hysterectomy
 c. Birth control pills
 d. Iron supplements

146. A patient is accidentally given the wrong medications by a nursing student. The nursing student apologized to the patient, but the patient does not speak English and has dementia. As the supervising nurse, which of the following is NOT an appropriate action?
    a. Call the nursing manager and the attending physician.
    b. Educate the nursing student about checking the medications and patient's identity prior to administration.
    c. Obtain a translator and discuss the error with the patient's family.
    d. Refrain from disclosing the incident unless negative sequelae develop.

147. A nurse comes on for the night shift and receives a patient who complained that he did not get his pain medications all day. The day nurse's notes reflect that no pain medications were given. Which of the following actions is the most appropriate?
    a. Tell the patient that the prior nurse forgot to give him medications.
    b. Give the patient extra pain medication to make up for it.
    c. Send the nurse an e-mail explaining that he/she did a poor job.
    d. Speak to the nurse manager about the issue.

148. A nursing colleague is assigned to take care of a local celebrity admitted to the hospital for an incomplete abortion. A news crew stops you outside of the hospital and asks for information about the patient. Which of the following is NOT an appropriate response?
    a. "No comment."
    b. "I was not responsible for the care of this patient."
    c. "She had an incomplete abortion and is in stable condition."
    d. "Only the patient or her power of attorney may give you that information."

149. A nursing student was walking through the hallway of the hospital and fell on a wet floor. The wet floor was caused by a leak in the ceiling. The maintenance worker was notified about the ceiling leak earlier, but never placed a caution sign. The goal of a root cause analysis would be to:
    a. Examine all of the contributing factors that led to the event.
    b. Identify the person/event to blame for the accident.
    c. Examine the efficacy of hospital hiring practices for its janitorial staff.
    d. Identify what caused the leak in the roof.

150. A nursing student asks his preceptor about Lantus's mechanism of action. Which of the following is the most appropriate response?
    a. "Its peak time is 8 to 12 hours."
    b. "Its peak time is 1 to 2 hours."
    c. "It is a short-acting insulin."
    d. "It is a continuous long-acting insulin."

Answers and Explanations

1. A: Chlamydia and gonorrhea are some of the few sexually transmitted diseases (STDs) that can be treated with antibiotics. Left untreated they can lead to pelvic inflammatory disease and infertility. Though some medical practitioners may believe that sex should be reserved until marriage, they should not push their personal beliefs on their patients. Patients should be educated about the spread of STDs and understand that one way to prevent the spread of diseases is by abstinence or practicing safe sex. Partners should always be informed once the diagnosis of an STD is made so they can be treated and prevent spreading the disease to others.

2. D: Calling the attending/resident/physician assistant on call is appropriate since the patient's ICP is high and the drain is not working. There may be a clot in the drain, which may or may not need to be flushed and which should not be done by the nurse. There are other reasons why a drain may not be working and it is up to the attending as to what the next step should be. A normal ICP should be between 0 and 20. A sustained ICP of 30 may cause permanent brain injury; monitoring it without calling an attending is inappropriate.

3. B: The use of restraints may worsen a decubitus ulcer because they keep the patient lying in one position. Frequent turning is important, allowing the patient's body weight to be distributed to other areas so that the pressure sore can heal. Air mattresses help alleviate the pressure that is placed on the body areas and wet-to-dry dressings help prevent against infection and promote healing.

4. C: Although increasing one's fluid intake is the most important way to help prevent kidney stones, there are food choices that may also help prevent reoccurrences. Foods such as lemons and limes can help dissolve existing stones. Kidney stones are usually made up of calcium oxalate which can be found in dairy, fruits such as apples and grapes, vegetables such as broccoli and turnips, beer, and several other foods. Those who suffer from kidney stones may find it advisable to limit foods high in calcium oxalate.

5. D: The nurse should call the physician to clarify the order. Lopressor is a beta blocker that can lower blood pressure and heart rate. If given an overdose of this medication, a patient may become dangerously hypotensive and may even die. It needs to be given in much smaller amounts in IV form since it is being injected directly into the bloodstream.

6. A: Bowel or bladder retention is not a risk factor for developing a decubitus ulcer. Bladder or bowel incontinence, however, is a risk factor since the skin is frequently in contact with feces and urine. Bacteria in the feces and/or urine may enter through a small break in the skin, causing an infection. Also if the skin is constantly covered in moisture the skin may become macerated and break down much more easily. Diabetics are much more prone to infections and are at risk for developing decubitus ulcers. Skin atrophy increases with increasing age, making it more susceptible to breakdown. Patients with peripheral vascular disease may have decreased sensation in their extremities and may not notice when they have a small wound on a part of their extremity. Also skin will heal poorly if the blood flow to the extremities is insufficient.

7. B: A chest x-ray should always be ordered after the placement of a nasogastric tube (NGT) to confirm that it is in the stomach and not in the lung. An abdominal x-ray would not be helpful. If the abdominal x-ray does not show the NGT, it tells the provider that it is not in the correct spot, but will not show where the NGT actually is. An abdominal ultrasound is used to examine visceral organs and vessels, which would not help identify an NGT placement. An EKG would not be helpful because it only monitors the heart.

8. C: Maintaining a patient's airway is of utmost importance. Fluid boluses help increase blood pressure, which increases the perfusion to vital organs and can be done in conjunction with or after maintaining the patient's airway. Obtaining a CT scan of the brain is important because it may help explain why the patient is hypotensive and lethargic (e.g., cerebral herniation may cause altered mental status and blood pressure changes). Emergent surgery may be needed to correct any intracranial pathology found. Antibiotics, if warranted, may be given once the patient is stabilized.

9. B: In accordance with The *Health Insurance Portability and Accountability Act* (HIPAA) healthcare providers may not give out patient information to anyone unless the patient gives permission to do so. In the event that patients are unconscious or lacking the capacity to give permission, healthcare providers may give information to the power of attorney or closest known family member (e.g., spouse, parent, child) as long as they provide documentation of their relationship status. Healthcare providers are not allowed to give information over the phone or in person to anyone other than the power of attorney unless the power of attorney grants permission. Healthcare providers may also not give the power of attorney's contact information to anyone.

10. C: Pneumovax 23 is a polyvalent pneumococcal vaccine, given prophylactically before surgery to prevent pneumococcal sepsis after splenectomy. Recombivax HB is a vaccine that protects against hepatitis. Attenuvax is a live, attenuated virus vaccine for immunization against measles (rubeola). Tetanus toxoid prevents tetanus (lockjaw) from *Clostridium tetani* infection after a puncture wound.

11. D: The nurse should call the attending to clarify the order. Lantus is a type of long-acting insulin and if the patient is being kept NPO he has no glucose intake to counteract the insulin therapy. This may result in dangerously low blood sugar levels. Since the patient has a subdural hematoma, he cannot have D5 in his IV fluids since this may result in cerebral edema. Generally Lantus is held prior to a procedure where the patient will be kept NPO, and the patient will be placed on regular insulin on a sliding scale.

12. B: Food, water, sleep, and excretion are the four fundamental needs or deficiency needs according to Maslow's hierarchy. These needs have to be fulfilled in order for a person to have a sense of peace and safety and be able to reach his/her full potential. Self-actualization is the highest-level need.

13. A: A line infection is generally not a common cause of post-operative fever within one week of surgery. A mnemonic for remembering the common causes of post-operative fever is the five Ws: **w**ind (atelectasis, aspiration, pneumonia), **w**ater (urinary tract infection), **w**alking (deep vein thrombus), **w**ound (wound infection), **w**hat the physician caused (drug fever, line infection). Wind is most likely to cause a fever POD 1–2, water is most likely to cause a fever POD 3–5, walking is the most likely to cause a fever POD 5–7, wound is the

most likely cause POD 5–9, and complications caused by the physician most likely cause a fever after the first week of surgery.

14. C: It is not advised that anyone recommend anti-depressant medications to a patient or patient's family member. If concerned about a psychological issue, a healthcare provider may make a referral to a psychiatrist and/or clinical psychologist who will then make his/her recommendations. Grief is very common after the loss of a loved one or a traumatic event, and medications, although usually beneficial, may not always be needed.

15. A: Diabetic ketoacidosis is caused by persistently high serum glucose which can present with dehydration, lethargy, urinary tract infection (caused by excessive sugar in the urine promoting bacterial growth), and fruity-scented breath. Correction includes aggressive IV fluid hydration and strict serum glucose management.

16. C: Sickle cell disease is an autosomal recessive disease that causes red blood cells to be abnormally shaped. This can cause chronic anemia, renal failure, cardiac arrest, splenomegaly, stroke, heart attack, and pulmonary embolus. There is no cure. Treatments include blood transfusions, pain medications, supplemental oxygen, and antibiotics or blood thinners/anti-platelet medications for secondary complications. It is diagnosed with a peripheral blood smear. A CBC may show nonspecific abnormalities, but is generally not diagnostic.

17. D: Bleeding is a common side effect of clopidogrel (Plavix) since it is an anti-platelet medication. It prevents the platelets from sticking together too readily and so helps prevent clot formation. Plavix is commonly prescribed after a patient has had a heart attack, cardiac surgery, or a stroke. The severity of the bleeding will determine whether or not the medication should be discontinued. Aspirin is another common anti-platelet medication.

18. B: Metabolic alkalosis. A blood pH higher than 7.45 and a bicarbonate level greater than 29 mEq/L confirm the diagnosis of metabolic alkalosis. A $PaCO_2$ greater than 45 mm/Hg indicates the patient's attempts at respiratory compensation.

19. B: The patient is in denial according to her response to her diagnosis. The five stages include denial, anger, bargaining, depression, and acceptance. Not all people go through all of the stages of grief, nor are they necessarily experienced in a particular order. In some cases, patients return to one or more stages several times until they are able to work through it.

20. D: Remaining hydrated is one of the most important recommendations that can be given to patients. If patients are in a hospital prior to the procedure, they should be on IV fluids. If they are doing the prep at home they should be told to drink water, Gatorade, and/or Jell-O to help prevent against dehydration, since they will be losing much of their body fluid due to the prep. They should never be advised to discontinue all of their medication. Sometimes medication does need to be discontinued prior to the procedure, but at other times it may be continued or the dosage may be adjusted depending on what the medication is and the condition it is treating. The patient should be ingesting fluids only; eating a pureed diet will interrupt the bowel prep and delay the procedure. Red foods or fluids should be avoided since they can mimic blood in the bowel which will impair the results of the colonoscopy.

21. C: Smoking should be avoided altogether since cigarette smoke can remain on someone's breath, skin, and clothing and therefore be inhaled when the affected person is nearby. Cigarette smoke is one of the most common triggers for an asthma attack. It is recommended that caregivers avoid smoking completely. Pet dander, strong perfumes/fragrances, and upper respiratory infections are also stimuli that can trigger an asthma exacerbation.

22. D: Steroids such as Decadron or prednisone can be used to treat a variety of disorders such as arthritis, dermatological conditions such as rosacea, and severe asthma, but can cause a multitude of complications if used long term such as diabetes, glaucoma, osteoporosis, hypertension, obesity, lowered immune system, and skin atrophy. Orange urine is a common side effect of Pyridium, which is used in conjunction with an antibiotic to treat urinary tract infections.

23. D: Hypomagnesemia. Crohn's disease is a type of autoimmune inflammatory bowel disease (IBD) that affects mostly the ileum and colon. However, the Crohn's patient may also have edema, redness, and dysfunction in the mouth, esophagus, and stomach. The Crohn's patient cannot absorb magnesium through the *lower* GI tract. Closely monitor your patient for hypomagnesemia. By contrast, potassium is affected by *upper* GI tract problems, such as vomiting.

24. D: Hypophosphatemia. Magnesium deficiency leads to impaired conservation of phosphate and, consequently, hypophosphatemia. Magnesium deficiency may also lead to hypocalcemia, hyponatremia, and hyperkalemia. Hypophosphatemia also occurs with inadequate nutrition.

25. C: Hand washing is the most important measure in preventing communicable diseases. Wearing gloves is important, but they may rip. If the gloves touch a contaminated surface and then touch someone's mouth or face, the gloves will not prevent against getting ill. However, wearing gloves in conjunction with hand washing is the most important way to prevent from getting ill and spreading disease to others. Wearing a face mask may help, but it does not fully prevent against spreading diseases. If someone's hands are contaminated and they touch their mouth or eyes, wearing a face mask will not prevent them from getting ill. Wearing goggles will prevent against splash of body fluids in one's eyes, but if one's hands are contaminated and the eyes are then touched, they will become contaminated as well.

26. D: Listeriosis is spread through contaminated food. Therefore, avoiding unpasteurized milk is recommended. It is also recommended to thoroughly wash produce, cook meat and fish prior to eating it, and to limit processed foods such as hot dogs and deli meats during pregnancy. Hot dogs and deli meats may be contaminated after they are cooked and prior to being packaged. Pregnant women infected with Listeria may only exhibit mild symptoms, but the illness may result in death of the fetus.

27. C: Gooseflesh and diarrhea
A drug with opiate antagonist properties may precipitate drug withdrawal in an opiate-dependent patient. Signs of opiate withdrawal include chills, sweats, gooseflesh, abdominal pain, muscle cramps, diarrhea, tearfulness, and irritability. Respiratory depression, nausea, and vomiting are adverse reactions to opiates, rather than signs of dependence. Seizures are a sign of sedative, hypnotic, or anxiolytic withdrawal.

28. A: Scabies infections are caused by mites burrowing underneath the skin in the web spaces of the fingers and toes. Topical medications such as permethrin cream can be used to treat infections. Pills are available for persistent infections refractory to topical treatment. Avoiding infected people and washing linens in hot water and bleach are other ways to treat the infection.

29. B: Trichomoniasis is least likely to cause cardiac arrest. It is a protozoal sexually transmitted disease commonly treated with Flagyl. There are twelve main causes of cardiac arrest (six Hs and six Ts): hypovolemia, hypoxia, hydrogen ions (acidosis), hyper/hypokalemia, hypothermia, toxins, tamponade, tension pneumothorax, thrombosis, thromboembolism, and trauma.

30. B: During the planning phase a nurse will develop his/her nursing care plan: how he or she will address the patient's medical problems according to the immediacy of each issue. The nurse will then develop a plan of desired outcomes to achieve based on the treatment plan. During the implementing phase the nurse will carry out his/her treatment plan and delegate tasks to others on the team. During the evaluating phase the nurse will monitor the patient's progress in response to treatment and further tailor or change the treatment plan accordingly if the results are unsatisfactory. During the diagnosing phase the nurse will create one or more diagnoses based on the patient's history and physical assessment.

31. C: Cystic fibrosis (CF) is an autosomal recessive genetic disorder that results in excessive accumulation of mucus in the GI and pulmonary tracts resulting in abdominal discomfort, chronic constipation, salty-tasting skin, poor appetite, fatigue, fever, and pancreatitis. Patients will experience a myriad of complications throughout their lifetime, but the most life threatening are persistent pulmonary infections such as pneumonia and progressive respiratory failure. The only treatment is symptomatic relief (i.e., skin emollients, nebulizers, stool softeners for constipation). The average lifespan is 30 to 40 years. Some patients have undergone lung transplants, but eventually the new lung will become diseased as well. Surgical intervention is used to prolong lifespan and will not cure the disease.

32. D: The patient is in the bargaining stage according to her response to her diagnosis. Patients hope that if they give up something, they can change their outcome. The five stages include denial, anger, bargaining, depression, and acceptance. Not all people go through all of the stages of grief nor are they necessarily experienced in a particular order. In some cases, patients return to one or more stages several times until they are able to work through it.

33. D: Tinnitus or ringing in the ears is not a typical symptom of asthma exacerbation. Asthma is a pulmonary disease that causes inflammation and bronchoconstriction of the airways. It may present with low-grade fever, wheezing, shortness of breath, nonproductive cough, and chest pain. It should be treated with supplemental oxygen and nebulizers, and in some cases steroids may be warranted.

34. B: Tonic-clonic or grand mal seizures present with generalized body tremors, tongue biting, diaphoresis, and/or urinary or bowel incontinence followed by a postictal period. The patient usually has no memory of the seizure itself. Petit mal is an outdated term for a cerebral seizure not exhibiting tonic-clonic movements. Absence seizures are more common

in children than adults. They can sometimes be misdiagnosed due to the unusual presentation of intermittently occurring blank staring episodes. A simple partial seizure presents with unilateral or generalized tremors, but the patient remains awake and alert throughout the entire seizure.

35. A: Compartment syndrome is a life-threatening condition which compromises the blood flow to the affected extremity. This could result in amputation if not treated emergently. Deep vein thrombosis (DVT) is dangerous because it puts a patient at higher risk for a pulmonary embolus (PE), but the development of a PE does not always occur. The presence of a DVT does not necessarily require emergent treatment. Muscle weakness and arthritis are potential complications of this patient's injury, but are not life threatening.

36. B: A repeat CT scan should be ordered in several hours to monitor the bleed. If the bleed increases in size then surgical intervention may be warranted. Since the patient has a bleed, anti-platelet medications such as aspirin and Plavix are contraindicated. Tissue plasminogen activator (tPA) is a very strong clot-busting medication given to patients with ischemic stroke or acute myocardial infarctions. Aspirin and Plavix can be given in cases of an ischemic stroke that is no longer in the tPA window or may be given to a patient who has a completed stroke. The tPA window is approximately three to four hours from time of witnessed onset of symptoms. The patient needs to be monitored in the hospital and should not be discharged home.

37. D: Celiac disease or celiac sprue is an immune reaction that damages the lining of the small intestine and prevents it from absorbing important nutrients. It presents as nausea, vomiting, diarrhea, and abdominal pain which occur after ingesting gluten-based products. The mainstay of treatment is to maintain a gluten-free diet to help prevent future exacerbations.

38. C: A patient with septic arthritis has an infection in the blood that is attacking a joint or joints. Obtaining blood cultures, lab work, getting a joint aspiration, and administering pain medications and IV antibiotics are several ways to help diagnose and treat this infection. NSAIDS may provide symptomatic relief, but would not help confirm the diagnosis. A 2D echo is an ultrasound of the heart; since the infection occurs in the joints, this would not help confirm the diagnosis. X-rays may be normal or may show nonspecific findings, but would not help confirm the diagnosis.

39. B: Food, water, sleep, and excretion are the four fundamental needs according to Maslow's hierarchy. These needs have to be fulfilled in order for a person to have a sense of peace and safety. The next level includes security of oneself and the safety of loved ones. The next level includes fulfillment of relationships with family members, friends, and intimacy with loved ones. Self-esteem is the second highest level, followed by the highest level of self-actualization.

40. B: Fish are very low in fiber and would not be recommended to patients who have a history of fecal impaction. High fiber foods such as bran, oatmeal, barley, raspberries, lentils, beans, broccoli, and peas would be recommended to help promote bowel movements and prevent fecal impaction in the future. Limiting narcotic medications and using stool softeners may also provide additional relief.

41. B: Fluid replacement

The primary treatment for a patient with hypernatremia is fluid replacement. The fluid of choice is determined by the cause of the imbalance. If the patient is hypovolemic, fluid replacement begins with normal saline solution and proceeds to 0.45 saline solution. If the cause of the hypernatremia is pure water loss, the fluid of choice is dextrose 5% in water. Giving sodium polystyrene sulfonate, which contains up to 10 g of sodium, would only increase the serum sodium level. Hypernatremia is associated with the use of diuretics, so avoid them. Activated charcoal does not absorb sodium and other small electrolytes.

42. A: An ileus is the most likely diagnosis for this patient's symptoms. It is the loss of peristalsis of the GI tract caused by disease, spinal cord injury, or following recent surgery. Symptoms include constipation, abdominal distention, nausea, and vomiting. Decompression with a nasogastric tube is usually the treatment. *C. difficile* colitis is a type of bacterial infection that causes severe profuse watery diarrhea, abdominal pain, and fever. It is common in patients who have been in the hospital for long periods of time and/or those who have been on long-term chemotherapy or antibiotics. Intussusception is a condition in which one part of the bowel folds in on itself and causes an obstruction. This is common in children. Symptoms include nausea, vomiting, lethargy, and red currant jelly stools. Toxic megacolon is a complication of *C. difficile* colitis. It is the pathologic distention of the colon caused by *C. difficile*, Crohn's disease, and ulcerative colitis. Signs and symptoms may include tachycardia, abdominal pain, abdominal distention, leukocytosis, and fever.

43. C: Calcium-rich foods such as yogurt, ice cream, milk, and cheese help prevent against gout exacerbations. Coffee and foods rich in Vitamin C such as oranges, strawberries, peppers, kiwi, and kale also help reduce a patient's risk. Patients should be counseled to refrain from or severely limit their intake of red meat, seafood, alcohol, and fructose. Medications used to prevent gout include allopurinol, NSAIDs, and steroids.

44. D: The patient with a known head trauma is experiencing a change in his neurological exam. The attending in charge of this patient's care should be made aware so he/she can decide the next step in intervention. Reassessing the exam in 30 minutes can delay the patient's treatment. A CT scan will most likely be ordered, but the attending should be made aware of the neurological change prior to ordering a CT scan. Percocet should be withheld from the patient for two reasons. First, Percocet is a narcotic that can further depress the neurological status and may hinder the ability to monitor whether or not this is a true change or it is due to the medication. Second, if the patient is lethargic he may aspirate on the medication, causing further complication to his condition.

45. B: Green leafy vegetables such as kale and spinach are high in vitamin K, which can act to reverse the effects of Coumadin. While patients do not necessarily need to cut them completely out of their diet, their intake of such foods should be monitored regularly. It is important to be consistent with the amount a person eats of these foods so that the INR can be monitored more effectively.

46. D: Exposure to extreme temperatures can cause an acute sickle cell crisis. Other common triggers can include hypoxia, dehydration, exposure to cigarette smoke, exposure to alcohol, and stress. Medical providers should encourage regular exercise with rest when becoming fatigued, adequate hydration, limiting tobacco, stress, and alcohol. Administration of fluids, pain medications, supplemental oxygen, and in some cases blood transfusions, are treatment modalities used during an acute sickle cell crisis.

47. C: Medications such as aspirin and Plavix act as anti-platelet medications. They prevent the platelets from sticking together too readily, which helps treat and prevent the formation of clots. Medications such as warfarin and Pradaxa act as blood thinners; warfarin and Pradaxa are not typically given for an acute myocardial infarction (MI). Medications like beta-blockers and narcotics are given to decrease workload on the heart and lower blood pressure by causing vasodilation. Morphine helps alleviate pain, which will also help lower blood pressure.

48. A: This patient may have pre-hypertension. Pre-hypertension is defined as a systolic blood pressure of 120 to 139 and diastolic blood pressure 81 to 89 on three consecutive visits four to six weeks apart. Medications can sometimes be avoided if patients take conservative measures to lower their blood pressure. However, since this patient is here for a wrist fracture, the elevated blood pressure may be due to pain. It should be recommended that the patient monitor his blood pressure for now and limit tobacco use.

49. C: A chest x-ray is one of the best diagnostic tests to confirm the presence of a pneumothorax or "dropped lung." It will show absence of lung markings and, if large enough, deviation of the trachea. An electrocardiogram may show some nonspecific abnormalities, but will not confirm the diagnosis. An echocardiogram is an ultrasound of the heart; it will not help confirm the diagnosis. Blood cultures play no role in diagnosing a pneumothorax.

50. A: Lasix is a diuretic which helps prevent and treat the presence of edema or excessive congestion. In cases of congestive heart failure, pulmonary edema, cirrhosis, and renal disease, fluid may collect in the body causing respiratory distress and/or extremity edema. Lasix inhibits sodium (and therefore water) from being absorbed in the kidneys, so it is excreted in the urine.

51. D: Lasix is a powerful diuretic which can cause hypokalemia. Patients discharged on Lasix may be given a potassium supplement or may be advised to supplement their diet with potassium-rich foods such as bananas, oranges, and spinach. The other choices provided are foods that are low in potassium and should be eaten in limited quantities for those who are taking Lasix.

52. B: The patient is at risk for developing diabetes. His fasting blood sugar and his HbA1c are borderline and he has a family history of diabetes. Anti-hyperglycemic medications such as Lantus and metformin at this point are unnecessary, but may be needed if his blood sugar cannot be controlled with diet and exercise. Rechecking an HbA1c in one week would be useless because it is a calculation of an average blood sugar level over a three-month period. This patient's HbA1c doesn't need to be checked for another three months. Levothyroxine is a medication used to treat hypothyroidism, not hyperglycemia.

53. D: This woman should be checked when she's 50 years old. The current recommendation in the United States is to get screened 10 years prior to the age of a first-degree relative who was diagnosed with colon cancer. If no risk factors are present then it is recommended to obtain a colonoscopy by 50 years of age.

54. A: A spiral CT scan or a CT angiogram (CTA) is the most diagnostic test for detecting the presence of a pulmonary embolus (PE). A ventilation perfusion scan may also be performed

- 34 -

but it is generally less diagnostic. It can only suggest the probability of a pulmonary embolism. The other drawback is that it cannot be done in patients on a ventilator. An echocardiogram is an ultrasound of the heart and plays no role in the workup of a PE. A chest x-ray may be completely normal or may show nonspecific abnormalities. However it is generally quicker to obtain than a CTA or ventilation perfusion scan, and may be ordered during the initial workup. An arterial blood gas may also be ordered in the initial workup to determine the severity of hypoxia.

55. C: Decreased red blood cell and platelet counts. You should expect to find a decreased red blood cell count and platelet count. Increased circulating catecholamines mobilize fatty acids, which leads to platelet aggregation. The reason red blood cells decrease is not clearly understood.

56. A: Turn the patient on his left side, with his head lower than his body. Chest pain and shortness of breath are associated with air embolism. Embolism is a serious complication that can occur with TPN administered through a central venous catheter. Turning the patient on his left side with his head lower than his body prevents the air from entering his pulmonary circulation. Calling a Code Blue and performing CPR are only appropriate if the patient experiences cardiac arrest. Do not stop TPN, unless air is visible in the tubing. The patient's signs and symptoms do not correlate with allergic reaction.

57. C: Monitor blood sugar levels because Carvedilol masks signs of hypoglycemia Beta-adrenergic blockers such as Carvedilol can mask a drop in blood sugar level, so the patient needs to monitor his blood sugar carefully. Carvedilol does not directly decrease perfusion, but may cause bradycardia, which could lead to decreased perfusion. All patients with diabetes should perform meticulous foot care because of neuropathy.

58. A: Tell the physician
A low-grade fever and calf swelling after recent surgery indicate probable deep vein thrombosis, so you should call the physician. Avoid manipulation (massaging the affected limb) or ambulation, as they could move the clot. Enforce bed rest until the presence of a clot is assessed through a venous Doppler series.

59. C: Condyloma acuminata or genital warts is a sexually transmitted disease. Factors such as birth-control usage, smoking, early age of first coitus, and multiple sexual partners increases the risk of contracting genital warts. There is no cure. The human papilloma virus (HPV) vaccine is available to help prevent genital warts.

60. B: Dwarfism occurs when there is a deficiency in growth hormone. Acromegaly will result in the presence of excessive growth hormone in an adult patient. Since adult patients have already stopped growing, growth hormone will cause bones to thicken and widen causing pain, weakness, and deformity. If excessive growth hormone occurs in children, gigantism will result since bones are still in the process of growing longitudinally. Diabetes occurs where there is either insufficient production of insulin (Type 2) or no insulin production due to an autoimmune reaction (Type 1).

61. B: The patient is suffering from acute alcohol intoxication. A normal alcohol level is less than 10; this patient's is 396. Treatment for acute alcohol intoxication is symptomatic relief. Anti-nausea medications, fluid hydration, and rest are the mainstays of therapy. Supplemental vitamins sometimes are given since chronic alcoholics are malnourished.

62. A: Pyridium is often given in conjunction with an antibiotic to help alleviate dysuria. The most common side effect of Pyridium is bright orange urine. Other common side effects may include headache and rash. While the decision to discontinue the medication must be based on the severity of the side effects, change in urine color should not be a reason to discontinue the medication. The urine will go back to its normal color once the medication course has been completed.

63. A: Dietary restrictions are an important part of controlling the neurological complications phenylketonuria (PKU) may cause. Patients with PKU are unable to break down phenylalanine, a common amino acid found in foods, most notably proteins. Patients with PKU must strictly adhere to diets low in phenylalanine. If the diagnosis is not made early or if patients are not compliant with their dietary restrictions, complications such as hyperactivity, seizures, and intellectual disability may occur.

64. B: Children less than six months of age are not recommended to get the influenza vaccine. Though almost everyone should get the flu vaccine every year, it is especially important for healthcare workers, immunocompromised individuals, people who are living in close quarters such as assisted-living facilities, hospitalized patients, and pregnant women.

65. C: Teach the patient to scan her visual field. Homonymous hemianopsia is the loss of one-half of the visual field in both eyes, either the right half or left half. Teach the patient to scan her visual field. Approaching the patient on her left side is ineffective because the loss is in both eyes. Homonymous hemianopsia does not affect hearing or swallowing.

66. C: Cardiac arrhythmias leading to heart failure are a common complication of thalassemia major. Thalassemia major is a rare genetic blood disorder in which the hemoglobin is defective. It causes mild to severe hemolytic anemia, which can commonly cause cardiac arrhythmias. The mainstays of treatment for thalassemia major are folate supplements and regular blood transfusions. In cases of severe disease, chelation therapy (removal of excess iron from the blood) and bone marrow transplants are necessary.

67. C: Pasta, baked goods, and processed foods lack iron and therefore should be avoided or severely limited in patients who have iron deficiency anemia. Foods high in calcium such as yogurt or broccoli have low iron content and impair iron absorption. Meat, eggs, and beans are obviously rich in protein and iron, but green leafy vegetables such as kale and spinach are also good sources of iron. Foods that have high vitamin C content such as oranges increase the body's ability to absorb iron.

68. D: A patient with hypovolemic shock should be placed in the Trendelenburg position. This involves the patient lying supine with the head of the bed tilted downward toward the floor, and the patient's legs may be either flexed or extended. This provides increased blood flow to the heart and other vital organs. The other positions involve the patient lying supine with the bed parallel to the ground.

69. B: Compartment syndrome is the swelling of muscle and surrounding tissue in response to an injury, which can swell to the point of cutting off the blood flow to the affected area. If not diagnosed quickly, it can result in loss of the limb. An arterial ultrasound Doppler, along with obtaining a history and physical examination, is the gold standard for diagnosing

compartment syndrome. It is easily obtainable, the test is resulted quickly, and there is minimal radiation involved. A CT scan may also be ordered, but it usually takes longer to obtain. MRIs are almost never ordered since not all hospitals have MRI machines and there is little information that an MRI can give that a CT scan cannot. X-rays are never ordered since they only show bones; vasculature is unable to be visualized on these films.

70. A: Intubating the patient and maintaining the airway is the crucial first step in managing this patient. When taking care of an unresponsive patient, think of the mnemonic ABC (Airway, Breathing, Circulation) as a way to prioritize things that need to be addressed. All three of these issues need to be addressed quickly in order to maximize the patient's chance for survival.

71. C: A nurse may try to find the air leak by gently clamping the chest tube momentarily along various sites using rubber-tipped clamps. You can destroy or partially ruin a chest tube by repeatedly stripping or "milking" it. A chest tube should never be pulled out unless the attending physician is present and authorizes the nurse to do so. Chest tubes are secured to the patient with sutures; in the event the chest tube is taken out, the sutures are cut and the chest tube is easily removed. By administering glue to the insertion site, you will make it incredibly difficult for the healthcare provider and very painful for the patient when the chest tube needs to be removed.

72. D: Lasix is a diuretic which decreases cerebral edema (thereby lowering the ICP) by causing fluid to shift out of the cranial vault into the circulation. It also interferes with the sodium transport, which slows the production of cerebrospinal fluid. Lantus is used to treat hyperglycemia. Levothyroxine is used to treat hypothyroidism. Lanoxin is used to treat cardiac *arrhythmias* such as atrial fibrillation.

73. B: "Have you had an upper respiratory tract infection recently?"
About 60% to 70% of clients with Guillain-Barré experience upper respiratory or GI viral infection 1 to 4 weeks before the symptoms of Guillain-Barré begin. The exact cause of Guillain-Barré syndrome is unknown, but it may be a cell-mediated immune response that attacks the peripheral nerves in response to a virus. The major pathological effect is segmental demyelination of the peripheral nerves, which destroys the myelin sheath of the nerve. Guillain-Barré is not a hereditary disorder. It is unrelated to viral exposure during foreign travel. It does not affect the clotting cascade.

74. B: Testicular torsion is a medical emergency. It occurs when the spermatic cord becomes twisted and blood flow to the testicle is severely diminished or absent, which may be precipitated by trauma. It presents with acute onset of pain and swelling of the affected testicle. A varicocele is an enlargement of the veins in the scrotum causing testicular aching and/or swelling to occur. The venous enlargement is usually due to faulty valves in the veins or compression of a neighboring vein disrupting blood flow in nearby veins. Palpation of the affected testicle is often described as feeling like "a bag of worms." A hydrocele is the collection of fluid around the testicle due to infection, malignancy, or unknown cause. It appears as a soft, usually painless mass on the testicle. This is not harmful and has no serious long-term complications. Testicular carcinomas present as hard, painless, fixed, solid testicular lesions.

75. C: Amiodarone, lidocaine, magnesium sulfate, vasopressin and/or epinephrine could be given during a code involving a patient with pulseless ventricular tachycardia. Dopamine is

used in patients with symptomatic bradycardia since dopamine increases one's heart rate. Since patients with ventricular tachycardia have an abnormally fast heart rate, dopamine should be avoided.

76. D: The patient can be given a full aspirin either by mouth or per rectum. The other option is to place a nasogastric tube (NGT) and give him his medications through the NGT. In either case the nurse should always clarify the order with the attending. A nurse should never skip a dose or cancel a medication without speaking to the attending first. If the patient has failed a swallow evaluation the nurse should not be feeding the patient at all. By giving the patient applesauce the nurse runs the risk of causing the patient to aspirate.

77. C: Tube feeds through a nasogastric tube (NGT) would be the preferred way to feed this patient. Since the patient has failed two swallow evaluations, choices A and B are contraindications since they can cause the patient to aspirate. Total parenteral nutrition (TPN) should be reserved for patients who suffer from severe chronic malnourishment, those who are on pressors, and those who have severe abdominal injuries or complications (e.g., pancreatitis or bowel fistula). TPN can cause liver failure, bowel atrophy, and infections. The general rule is that if the gut works, use it.

78. D: Bipolar disorder is a psychiatric disorder featuring episodes of extreme happiness and energy followed by periods of depression. Anorexia nervosa is an eating disorder, much more common in girls than boys and most common in adolescents, which involves purposely starving oneself in order to lose weight. Bulimia nervosa is an eating disorder, much more common in girls than boys and most common in adolescents, which involves periods of binging followed by periods of fasting in order to lose weight. Generalized anxiety disorder is a psychiatric disorder causing a person to feel anxious or nervous most or all of the time with no known cause.

79. A: The supine position is best for a patient who is suffering from a headache post lumbar puncture. This is because the cerebrospinal fluid bathes the brain in fluid, which may alleviate or at least improve the headache. All of the other positions involve the patient sitting up or having the head raised, which will exacerbate the headache and increase the risk for developing a subdural hematoma and/or seizure.

80. D: Adenosine may be given to a patient in supraventricular tachycardia. Norvasc is used in the treatment of hypertension, not tachycardia. Its use is not indicated in ACLS protocol. Tylenol may be used for pain or inflammation, but is not part of ACLS protocol. Morphine is a narcotic medication that can slow the heart rate, but is not used in ACLS protocol.

81. A: The North American Nursing Diagnosis Association International (NANDA-I) taxonomy system is used to standardize nursing diagnoses worldwide. It is also used as a way to universally define certain medical conditions as well as identify risk factors that are associated with certain pathologies.

82. B: Placement of an orthopedic boot is the most appropriate treatment for foot drop. For severe cases, surgery may be indicated. Foot drop causes the foot to be extended with limited or no ability to dorsiflex; it is most often caused by trauma or disease affecting the muscles or the nerves. Keeping the foot propped up on the pillow or massaging the foot would be ineffective treatments since the foot itself is not being treated. Placement of an

elastic stocking would help with circulation, but foot drop is not caused by a circulatory disorder.

83. D: Increasing one's calcium intake is advice usually given to someone with osteopenia or osteoporosis. Osteopenia is lower than average bone mineral density, but is not as severe as osteoporosis. Raynaud's disease is caused by the body's abnormal response to cold weather and to stress. A way to prevent or limit the severity of an exacerbation is to avoid cold exposure as much as possible by dressing in warm layers. Limiting one's intake of red meat and alcohol is advice usually given to someone with gout. Increasing one's fluid intake is advice usually given to someone with nephrolithiasis.

84. C: The costovertebral angle (CVA) is defined as the area where the twelfth rib joins the spine. If palpation causes costovertebral angle tenderness (CVAT) then a kidney infection is likely present since the kidneys are located just below the twelfth ribs. Cholecystitis or appendicitis may be suspected if the patient had right-sided or epigastric abdominal pain. A small bowel obstruction may be present if a patient has constipation, diffusely distended and tender abdomen, and has persistent nausea and/or vomiting.

85. B: Reynold's pentad is Charcot's triad (RUQ pain, fever, jaundice) that occurs with shock (hypotension) and altered mental status. This is seen in patients with ascending cholangitis. In cases of patients with Charcot's triad, biliary drainage should be performed once the patient is stabilized. When a patient presents with Reynold's pentad, a biliary drainage should be performed emergently.

86. B: Permethrin is used to treat scabies and plays no role in the treatment of cystic fibrosis. Cystic fibrosis (CF) is an autosomal recessive genetic disorder that results in excessive accumulation of mucus in the GI and pulmonary tracts resulting in abdominal discomfort from chronic constipation, dry salty-tasting skin, poor appetite, fatigue, fever, and pancreatitis. The only treatment is symptomatic relief (i.e., nebulizer treatments, emollients, stool softeners for constipation). Antibiotics are used for infections.

87. C: Although all medical professionals are bound by HIPAA (Health Insurance Portability and Accountability Act) which ensures patient privacy, there are instances where the medical professional may share a patient's information. If a patient threatens to injure themselves or others, a medical professional may reach out to local authorities or family members to warn them of the patient's potential plans in order to ensure the safety of the patient and others.

88. D: After a recent femur fracture a patient should not be riding a motorcycle since high speed collisions are the number one cause of femur fractures. These collisions commonly involve motorcycles, though they can also occur during a car accident. Most patients are encouraged to participate in physical therapy and to ambulate early in the post-operative period to help prevent muscle wasting, pressure ulcers, and blood clots. Three months after the event the patient should be able to perform self-care activities since the cast and/or external fixator(s) should be removed by then.

89. A: Patients who are taking ACE inhibitors have approximately a 10 percent chance of developing hyperkalemia. A patient with chronic renal insufficiency may have hyperkalemia at baseline since the kidneys are responsible for filtering excess potassium from the body. Further evidence that the patient has hyperkalemia is the appearance of peaked T waves on

the EKG. Since the patient has chronic renal insufficiency, the BUN and creatinine should be mildly elevated. Variations exist between labs, but a normal BUN is 12–22, normal creatinine is 0.9–1.1, and normal potassium level is 3.5–5.1. Choice A is the only one that has abnormally high values for all three labs.

90. A: Lovenox or heparin are generally used to treat superficial vein thromboses (SVTs). Coumadin is generally not indicated unless multiple clots are present and/or if a patient has an underlying hypercoagulable disorder. Compression stockings are contraindicated in those with a DVT/SVT since they can propagate the clot. They would also not be used since compression stockings are used for lower extremities only. Warm compresses are not indicated unless there is a secondary infection.

91. D: A lumbar puncture plays no role in the treatment of thalassemia major. Thalassemia major is a genetic blood disorder that results in moderate to severe hemolytic anemia. Folate supplements are commonly used, but may not be sufficient enough. Since patients have an abundance of iron in their blood, chelation therapy is often used in conjunction with blood transfusions.

92. A: Acromegaly is not a sign of Cushing's disease. Acromegaly results from the presence of excessive growth hormone in an adult patient. Since adult patients have already stopped growing, growth hormone will cause bones to thicken and widen causing pain, weakness, and deformity. Cushing's disease is due to the presence of excessive cortisol causing unintentional weight gain, striae, a fat pad or buffalo hump on the posterior neck, facial swelling, and osteoporosis.

93. D: Ativan is a benzodiazepine which causes mild to moderate sedation. Since patients with acute alcohol intoxication already have a depressed mental status, medications such as Ativan should be avoided. Vitamins such as thiamine, magnesium, and folic acid are frequently administered to alcoholic patients since they are usually chronically malnourished and suffer from electrolyte imbalances due to their addiction. Zofran is an antiemetic medication that prevents and alleviates nausea and vomiting.

94. C: The Joint Commission defines a sentinel event as an unexpected injury or complication, which may or may not cause the death of the patient, not due to the patient's primary diagnosis. Leaving a surgical instrument in the patient's head causing a brain abscess is not caused by the patient's stroke. The instrument left inside of the patient's head is the sentinel event. The brain abscess is the complication. The ischemic stroke is the original diagnosis. The hemorrhagic stroke is an expected risk of tPA administration. Tissue plasminogen activator (tPA) is a very strong clot-busting medication given to patients with stroke or acute myocardial infarctions. After being given this medication patients generally should not receive blood thinners, anti-platelet medications, or lines since their risk of bleeding is very high.

95. A: A pneumothorax or "dropped lung" can sometimes be monitored with serial chest x-rays and oxygenation status if it is small. Moderate or large defects should be corrected with placement of a chest tube. Since this condition is painful, pain medications such as narcotics may be used. Warm compresses play no role in treatment.

96. D: Gastroesophageal reflux disease (GERD) is caused by the lower esophageal sphincter closing improperly, which allows stomach acid to escape into the esophagus. Medications

such as NSAIDs may erode the lining of the stomach. Esomeprazole is a proton pump inhibitor which causes the stomach to produce less acid. Therefore less acid is available to be released into the esophagus and/or to erode the stomach lining. Taking esomeprazole will alleviate or partially alleviate symptoms and damage done to the esophageal mucosa.

97. C: The number one cause of pelvic inflammatory disease (PID) is venereal disease, most notably gonorrhea and chlamydia. Untreated sexually transmitted diseases may lead to pelvic inflammatory disease, which is the leading primary preventable cause of infertility. Approximately 10 to 15 percent of PID cases are caused by illnesses such as appendicitis, or pelvic procedures such as dilation and curettage, abortion, or childbirth. PID may be caused by a pelvic procedure, such as the removal of an ectopic pregnancy, or PID may cause an ectopic pregnancy to occur.

98. D: Reverse Trendelenburg. The patient's head is upright in the reverse Trendelenburg position and down in the Trendelenburg position. Both positions protect the spinal cord because the bed surface is flat, but reverse Trendelenburg also protects the patient's airway by allowing secretions to drain out. High Fowler's bends the spine, so do not use it until the radiologist rules out spinal cord injury. A flat bed allows spine stability but does not protect the patient's airway.

99. D: Caffeine can cause insomnia, abdominal cramping, diarrhea, and may cause food cravings. It should generally be avoided before and during one's menses. Exercise has been shown in numerous studies to limit feelings of depression and provide extra energy during the day. Eating nutritious meals and snacks throughout the day can help regulate blood sugar, which can curb binge eating, food cravings, and mood swings due to hyperglycemia or hypoglycemia. Birth control pills can better regulate hormones, which may alleviate or at least partially reduce mood swings and depression caused by premenstrual syndrome.

100. D: Many cases of cervical cancer are caused by the human papilloma virus (HPV). Limiting one's sexual partners can decrease one's exposure to HPV and can decrease the risk of developing cervical cancer. Regular Pap smears and gynecological examinations can help detect any anomalies early. Venereal/sexually transmitted disease screening plays little role since HPV is not treatable. The use of diaphragms plays no role in the development or prevention of cervical cancer. Alcohol intake does not increase one's risk significantly.

101. B: Beriberi is caused by a thiamine deficiency primarily seen in developing or underdeveloped countries. Symptoms may include muscle weakness or paralysis due to damaged nerves, heart failure, pleural effusion, encephalopathy, seizures, decreased reflexes, as well as a multitude of other complications. Some of these complications may be permanent if the thiamine deficiency is not corrected quickly.

102. A: Diabetes mellitus is the insufficient production of insulin resulting in hyperglycemia. Maintaining an ideal body weight and limiting the amount of sugar and processed foods can help prevent the development of the disease. Increasing one's thiamine intake would help prevent beriberi. Decreasing alcohol intake would help those who are chronic alcoholics or those with gout. Increasing iron intake will help those with anemia.

103. A: In the awake, alert patient with a caretaker at the bedside, who is asymptomatic, other interventions should be considered first before giving D5W. Eating lunch, especially

consuming a short acting carb to raise the blood sugar now, and a long acting carb to help sustain blood sugar levels and prevent rebound hypoglycemia is advisable. However, if the patient in the situation had depressed mental status, juice should not be given since the patient would be at risk for aspiration. The blood sugar should be rechecked to make sure that it is rising appropriately. Advising the patient to avoid rising and walking will help the patient stay safe from falls. Change in mental status could indicate that the patient's blood sugar is getting lower and further intervention is needed.

104. C: The patient does not need to be on bed rest. Reasonable physical activity as tolerated is encouraged in both inpatient and outpatient settings for stroke patients to help them improve their range of motion, ambulation, and strength. Recommending bed rest will only exacerbate their residual deficits caused by the stroke and increase the risk for deep vein thromboses, decubitus ulcers, and atelectasis.

105. B: This patient is having a transfusion reaction. The transfusion should be stopped immediately before performing any interventions. You may administer Benadryl for pruritus and for the rash, and Tylenol may be given for fever and pain. Steroids may also be given to help decrease inflammation. Since the patient is having chest pain, an EKG would also be an appropriate intervention.

106. D: The transfusion reaction was caused by the patient receiving the incorrect blood type. Any time a patient is receiving medication, blood products, or is undergoing a procedure, the patient's identity and blood type should be verified by at least two nurses. The blood product should also be examined to make sure it has the correct name and blood type. The Joint Commission defines a sentinel event as an unexpected injury or complication, which may or may not cause the death of the patient, not due to the patient's primary diagnosis. The pulmonary embolus is an expected potential complication of having sickle cell disease. Although the patient developed epistaxis from the Coumadin and heparin, it is an expected potential complication of anticoagulation medications. The patient developed a transfusion reaction due to human error and not from her primary diagnosis.

107. A: Hypervolemia, hypertension, and hemodilution, otherwise known as "triple H" therapy of subarachnoid hemorrhages, is the gold standard of treatment. Keeping a patient's blood pressure elevated, maintaining hypervolemia through blood transfusions and hemodilution through aggressive fluid hydration helps prevent further complication from vasospasm such as stroke.

108. A: An ileus is the impaired peristalsis of the gastrointestinal tract following a surgery or accompanying certain diseases. It may present with nausea, vomiting, constipation, and distended abdomen. Trickle feeds, bowel regimen medications such as Colace and senna, and anti-emetic medications are the mainstays of therapy for an ileus.

109. A: There are three stages in the nurse-client therapeutic relationship: orientation, exploration, and termination. In the first stage the nurse and client establish limitations, boundaries, trust, and rapport. In the second stage the nurse and client should be able to identify problems or issues and potential solutions to those issues. The nurse may offer assistance or teach the client coping mechanisms in order to face some of the issues. The nurse may assume different roles in order to help the client deal with the stressful situation he or she is facing. In the last phase, the relationship is terminated upon discharge or

transfer. The goal of the third stage is the resolution of the client's issues and/or achieving acceptance of the problems and ways to cope with them.

110. B: Bleeding is a common side effect of blood thinners such as Coumadin or Pradaxa or anti-platelet medications like aspirin or Plavix. Ototoxicity is one of the most common side effects of the <u>aminoglycosides</u>, such as gentamicin. Cough is one of the most common side effects of ACE inhibitors. Liver failure can be caused by a number of medications.

111. B: The **Omnibus Budget Reconciliation Act (OBRA),** also known as the Nursing Home Reform Act of 1987, mandates the minimum standards of care for nursing home facilities. These mandates cover aspects of care such as addressing each resident's medical, social, and emotional needs; preventing the decline of the ability to perform basic activities of daily life and providing assistance if those abilities do decline; safety measures; and other standards that keep nursing home residents reasonably healthy and comfortable.

112. D: Nexium and Plavix should never be taken together since Nexium blunts the effects of Plavix. Nexium blocks an enzyme in the body that turns Plavix into its active form. This can increase the risk of a patient developing an adverse event such as stroke or heart attack. If a patient who needs Plavix is taking Nexium, this should be switched to a histamine-2 blocker such as Pepcid.

113. C: Sjögren's syndrome is an autoimmune disease that causes insufficient production of saliva and mucus in the body. The most common complaints of patients include eye, nasal, and vaginal dryness. In order to help alleviate these symptoms, medical professionals should recommend the use of lubricants, nasal sprays, and eye drops.

114. C: Superficial vein thrombosis (SVT) or deep vein thrombosis (DVT) is usually caused by lack of physical activity; bed rest will only cause more clots to develop. Subcutaneous heparin or Lovenox are used as treatment and prevention of SVTs and DVTs. If the patient is at high risk and there are no contraindications, Coumadin may be started. In cases where Coumadin is contraindicated, placement of an inferior vena cava filter (IVCF) may be indicated. If a patient is diagnosed with a clot, repeat ultrasound Dopplers should be ordered to monitor the progression of the clot.

115. A: Status epilepticus is a condition in which a patient continually seizes without break. Finger sweeps are contraindicated because the patient can bite down on the examiner's finger causing injury or amputation. The patient should be placed in reverse Trendelenburg position to maintain a patent airway; if the patient develops hypoxia, supplemental oxygen is recommended. Anti-seizure medications such as Vimpat, Dilantin, or Keppra are warranted.

116. A: Lorazepam is a benzodiazepine. Benzodiazepines cause sedation, so they are commonly used as treatment for anxiety disorders, phobia disorders, and seizures. Lantus is an anti-hyperglycemic medication commonly used in diabetic patients. Levoxyl is a synthetic thyroid hormone medication used in patients who have hypothyroidism. Lopressor is a beta-blocker which is used to decrease heart rate and blood pressure. *It is used for treatment of hypertension, atrial fibrillation, heart failure, and acute myocardial infarction.*

117. D: Lexapro is used to treat generalized anxiety disorder, depression, post-traumatic stress disorder, and other psychiatric conditions. Decadron is a type of steroid used to treat inflammatory reactions such as localized skin reactions and asthma. Lantus is used to treat those with hyperglycemia. Permethrin is used to treat infections caused by scabies.

118. D: Destroy intestinal organisms that break down proteins to ammonia
Hepatic encephalopathy is characterized by elevations of ammonia levels in the brain and cerebrospinal fluid. Ammonia is produced in the GI tract when bacteria break down protein. Neomycin reduces ammonia-forming bacteria in the intestinal tract. Neomycin is not absorbed into the circulation, so it exerts a powerful effect on intestinal bacteria. The other options do not correctly explain neomycin's use.

119. D: RhoGAM is administered to prevent hemolytic disease of the newborn, or Rhesus disease. This can result in jaundice, heart failure, hepatosplenomegaly, and fetal death. It is caused by maternal antibodies of a Rhesus negative mother that attack a Rhesus positive fetus. The positive Rhesus factor is regarded by the mother's body as a foreign antigen, so the mother's antibodies attack the fetus. RhoGAM is an immune globulin that depresses the mother's immune system temporarily so that it does not recognize the positive Rhesus fetus.

120. A: If a needle-stick injury occurs, the most important first step is to scrub out and immediately irrigate or wash the wound with soap and water. This is done not only for the nurse's safety, but also for the safety of the patient. The patient should be notified of the incident once he/she has awakened from anesthesia. Employee health and the nursing supervisor should be immediately notified. The nurse with the needle-stick injury should report to the emergency department so blood can be drawn for virology.

121. D: Ask the patient to extend her arm and hyperextend her hand
Asterixis is a flapping hand tremor that is a classic sign of hepatic failure. To check for asterixis, ask the patient to extend her arm and hyperextend her fingers toward the ceiling. Observe if the patient can maintain this position or if her fingers begin to tremble. Asterixis is a hand tremor only, testing the feet, having the patient squat, and measuring the abdominal girth are inappropriate measures.

122. C: The patient should be allowed to drink small sips of water to try and clear her throat. The patient is able to cough which means that her airway is not completely obstructed. Finger sweeps should never be performed because you increase the risk of pushing the object further into the airway. Since the patient is still coughing, she is able to move air in and out of her lungs. Performing back slaps or abdominal thrusts is indicated only if there is a complete obstruction.

123. A: Though Dilantin may be an appropriate medication to be given during an acute seizure, a nurse should never give a medication without an order from an attending physician, resident, or licensed independent practitioner (LIP). In order to prevent aspiration, the patient should be placed on his side, and if the patient had been eating, food should be cleared from the mouth. The attending should be called immediately so orders can be given to treat the patient. The family should be kindly asked to leave the room so the patient can be treated more effectively. Once the patient is stabilized the family members can be brought back into the room and be given updates on how the patient was treated and his response to the treatment.

124. A: Chvostek's sign. Chvostek's sign is seen with hypocalcemia, which occurs in acute pancreatitis as calcium binds to areas of fat necrosis in the pancreas. Check for Chvostek's sign by tapping over the facial nerve and observing facial twitching. Trousseau's sign also indicates hypocalcemia. Acute pancreatitis usually causes hypoactive bowel sounds, and the serum glucose level is increased. Shortness of breath usually is not seen in alcoholic pancreatitis.

125. D: Gastroesophageal reflux disease (GERD) is caused by the lower esophageal sphincter closing improperly, which allows stomach acid to escape into the esophagus. Any acidic foods/drinks such as grapefruit, oranges, lemons, limes, grapes, and wine should be avoided. Fatty or fried foods can also cause an acid reflux exacerbation and should generally be limited or avoided altogether. Oatmeal helps absorb acidity and helps prevent acid reflux. Other foods that help those with acid reflux include tea, fennel, green leafy vegetables, watermelon, potatoes, and cereal.

126. D: Have the patient lie in a lateral decubitus knee-bent position
Lying on the side with knees bent reduces the amount of tension on abdominal muscles and may provide some pain relief. Lying supine or standing would increase abdominal tension and pain. Food, heat, and activity also increase pain.

127. D: Frequent repositioning. The liver synthesizes coagulation factors and converts ammonia to urea. Hepatic failure is indicated by this patient's laboratory values. Liver failure increases serum ammonia levels and bleeding times, which can cause tissue breakdown. Frequent repositioning helps to avoid liver destruction. Liver patients should receive mouth care several times a day and be placed in a quiet environment. In addition, most liver patients have a nasogastric tube in place, due to abdominal distention and vomiting.

128. D: Tonometry measures intraocular pressure, which helps to diagnose intraocular abnormalities such as glaucoma. Calorimetry helps measure heat given off by the physical and chemical breakdown of a substance. A fluorescein screen is an eye test that diagnoses whether or not a corneal abrasion or tear is present. Spirometry is a pulmonary function test that helps evaluate lung function.

129. B: Metabolic acidosis. Total parenteral nutrition may lead to hyperchloremia, causing bicarbonate levels to decrease, which in turn leads to metabolic acidosis. Hypokalemia, hyperglycemia, hyponatremia, and hypophosphatemia are also common with total parenteral nutrition.

130. C: Administering diuretics, as prescribed, and maintaining sodium restriction
Ascites is fluid accumulation in the abdominal cavity from inflammation of the liver. Administering diuretics and maintaining sodium restriction best relieves ascites. Supplemental oxygen does not change the underlying problem of ascites. The patient would breathe best in semi-Fowler's position, not supine position. A low protein and fat-restricted diet is appropriate for hepatic failure, but does not affect ascites.

131. B: A patient with a terminal disease or injury with severely depressed mental status may be made CMO by the family/power of attorney, which allows the healthcare team to assist in the process of dying while ensuring that the patient is made comfortable. This

entails withholding life-saving measures/medications, supplemental oxygen, CPR, IV fluids, and tube feeds/food. Since the patient cannot be asked how much pain/discomfort he is in, the healthcare team assesses the patient's discomfort by his vital signs. A patient is usually placed on narcotic pain medications and/or sedatives (depending on the hospital protocol and the state in which the hospital is located), which will be given if the patient develops tachycardia, tachypnea, or becomes hypertensive.

132. C: A patient should be able to urinate normally after surgery; this patient may be suffering from urinary retention, and a bladder scan should be ordered after notifying the attending physician. It is normal to have abdominal pain upon coughing or sneezing after undergoing abdominal surgery since these actions can increase intra-abdominal pressure. A nurse may suggest that the patient hold a pillow to her abdomen to help alleviate the discomfort. A patient's appetite may take a few days to return to normal after abdominal surgery; a nurse may suggest that she eat/drink as tolerated and limit fatty or greasy foods since these can further exacerbate abdominal discomfort. Abdominal pain is normal after abdominal surgery as long as it is not severe, intractable pain.

133. A: Ensure proper fluid and electrolyte replacement. Small bowel obstruction causes profuse vomiting, which leads to fluid and electrolyte loss. It is essential to correct electrolyte loss before surgery. There is no indication that an ileostomy is required. The physician obtains informed consent, not the nurse. TPN will most likely be used later, but is not as important as preventing shock from fluid loss or electrolyte depletion.

134. D: The patient is developing "Red Man Syndrome" which is a hypersensitivity reaction to Vancomycin. It is not considered a true allergy since it is generally due to the drug being infused too quickly rather than being due to the drug itself. The first step is to discontinue the infusion. Next, the patient may be treated with NSAIDs, Benadryl, or steroids, and/or antiemetics for additional relief. If the drug is to be given again in the future, the patient should be given NSAIDs, Benadryl, and/or steroids prior to the antibiotic being infused. Also, the drug should be infused at a very slow rate. Administering supplemental oxygen in this case is unnecessary since the patient's vital signs are stable.

135. B: The western blot test would confirm the diagnosis of HIV/AIDS. The Mantoux tuberculin skin test diagnoses tuberculosis. The RPR will help diagnose those who have syphilis. The India ink test would be positive in those who are suffering from a cryptococcal infection. Cryptococcal infections are common in patients with depressed immune function, such as AIDS patients, but the presence of the infection is not diagnostic for AIDS.

136. A: Although the patient's HDL (a.k.a. "good" cholesterol) is very good, both the LDL and triglyceride levels are high, so the patient would benefit from a statin. In women an HDL level less than fifty and in men a level less than forty increases the risk for having a stroke or heart attack. A triglyceride level less than 150 is considered normal. A triglyceride level above 200 is considered high and warrants medical management. An LDL level of less than 100 is considered normal. A level above 160 is considered high and warrants medical management.

137. B: Respiratory distress syndrome (ARDS). ARDS can occur in acute pancreatitis as a result of hypoperfusion and shock. Hypocalcemia and diabetes mellitus, not hypercalcemia and diabetes insipidus, may occur in pancreatitis. Pericarditis is not associated with pancreatitis.

138. D: Diabetes mellitus is a disease wherein an insufficient production of insulin by the pancreas causes hyperglycemia. Symptoms include polyuria, polyphagia, polydipsia, weakness, and fatigue. Ordering a hemoglobin A1c (or HbA1c) can not only make the diagnosis, but is also used to monitor the patient's response to treatment.

139. D: Phytonadione (Vitamin K) is necessary to produce prothrombin. Heparin increases the risk of bleeding. Packed red blood cells increase the oxygen carrying capacity of the blood but do not prevent bleeding. Protamine sulfate antagonizes heparin and has no effect on prothrombin.

140. A: Hashimoto's disease is an autoimmune disease causing hypothyroidism. If hypothyroidism is left untreated it can cause bradycardia, unintentional weight gain, hair loss, and permanent neurological deficit. There is no way to cure Hashimoto's disease, but exogenous thyroid hormone may be taken daily to prevent complication.

141. A: MRI is the best test to diagnose osteomyelitis. Osteomyelitis is an infection and inflammation of the bone. X-rays may be diagnostic, but in some cases they may be normal or show nonspecific findings. The use of ultrasound and EKG are not helpful in making the diagnosis. Once the diagnosis is made, administration of IV antibiotics is initiated.

142. C: No intervention is needed if both the mother and baby are Rh negative. The Rh factor is an antigen that may or may not be attached to one's blood cells. Those who have a positive blood type (A+, B+, O+, AB+) have the antigen. Those who have a negative blood type do not have the antigen and are Rh negative. If a mother is Rh negative and her unborn child is Rh positive, RhoGAM needs to be administered. RhoGAM is an injection that suppresses the mother's immune response to the Rh positive baby, which can help prevent hemolytic disease of the newborn. Antibiotics are unnecessary because it is a blood incompatibility issue, not an infection. An ultrasound would be ineffective for concerns regarding Rh factor.

143. B: The patient has trichomoniasis. It is caused by a protozoan infection of the genitourinary tract. It is a sexually transmitted disease which can cause green frothy discharge from the penis or vagina, dysuria, pain with sexual intercourse, and strong, foul vaginal odor. The treatment of choice is metronidazole. The patient should be advised to maintain abstinence or practice safe sex.

144. A: D5W contains 5% dextrose in water, which is a hypotonic solution. It draws water out of the circulation and into the cells. This is a problem in patients with intracerebral hemorrhages, vasogenic edema, and/or patients with high intracranial pressure because this can exacerbate their condition. D5W should never be ordered in these patients. The other options are either isotonic solutions (normal saline and lactated Ringer's) or hypertonic solutions (3% NaCl) which are acceptable to use in brain injury patients.

145. B: Fibroids are benign growths which may cause dysmenorrhea, menorrhagia, pain with sexual intercourse, abdominal cramping, and urinary frequency. NSAIDs, birth control pills, and iron supplements are the initial treatments. For symptoms refractory to conservative therapy or for severe bleeding, surgery may be recommended. Since the patient is newly diagnosed and because she is so young, hysterectomy would not be considered the initial treatment.

146. D: Full disclosure is of the utmost importance not only because it is the ethical thing to do, but also for legal purposes. Even though the patient does not speak English and has dementia, the family member(s) or power of attorney should be notified of the error whether or not negative sequelae develop. The nursing student should be educated about checking and rechecking the patient's identity (by room number and by hospital bracelet) and the medications that are due to be given. The attending physician and the nurse manager should also be made aware so they can also monitor for negative reactions to the medication.

147. D: Speaking to the nurse manager privately about the issue so she or he can investigate it further is the most appropriate action. Perhaps the patient did not complain to his nurse that he was in pain and that is why she or he did not give the medications. Even if the patient did complain to the nurse about his pain and the nurse did not provide adequate pain management, it is unprofessional to discuss the nurse's behavior with the patient. It is illegal and unethical to give patients extra medication that is not ordered for them. It is unprofessional to send emails to colleagues regarding their performance.

148. C: In accordance with The *Health Insurance Portability and Accountability Act* (HIPAA) healthcare providers may not give out patient information to anyone unless the patient gives permission to do so. In the event that the patient is unconscious or lacking the capacity to give permission, the healthcare provider may give information to the power of attorney or closest known family member (i.e., spouse, parent, child) as long as documentation of the relationship status is provided. Healthcare providers are not allowed to give information over the phone or in person to anyone other than the power of attorney unless the power of attorney grants permission.

149. A: The goal of root cause analysis is to examine all of the factors leading to the event that allowed an accident or error to occur. The goal is not to blame one particular person or event. It attempts to look at ways in which practices, policies, and/or behaviors can be modified or changed in order to help ensure that the accident/error does not happen in the future.

150. D: Lantus is a type of long-acting continuous insulin. It is useful in patients who do not experience intermittent hypoglycemia. It should not be used in patients who are going to be undergoing surgery and need to be NPO, since Lantus can cause their blood sugar to drop dangerously low. The Lantus dose may need to be lower in those with hepatic or renal impairment since the drug will be metabolized slower and end up in the patient's system longer than intended.

Practice Questions

1. According to Maslow's hierarchy, after physiological needs are met which of the following needs are the second-most important?
    a. Safety/security
    b. Sexual intimacy
    c. Self esteem
    d. Self actualization

2. Your patient had a complete colectomy with an ileostomy. Identify the nursing action that is most important for this patient:
    a. Monitor the patient for fluid and electrolyte imbalances
    b. Administer proteolytic enzymes to aid digestion of fats and proteins
    c. Use warm tap water irrigations to prevent stool retention
    d. Use mild antidiarrheal medications to prevent nutritional losses

3. Your patient is scheduled to receive hemodialysis at 10:00 a.m. and has several medications ordered at 9:00 a.m. Choose the most appropriate action:
    a. Give the medications at 9:00 am
    b. Call the physician for further instructions
    c. Hold all medications until dialysis is complete
    d. Give the medications that will be retained, and hold those that would be dialyzed out.

4. Your patient's diagnosis is prerenal failure. Identify the nursing intervention that is top priority for him:
    a. Administer antibiotics, as prescribed
    b. Administer I.V. fluid boluses, as prescribed
    c. Reposition frequently
    d. Provide frequent oral hygiene

5. A patient is admitted for a stroke. The nurse notices that the patient has developed contracture of the arm. Which of the following is NOT an appropriate intervention?
    a. Daily massage
    b. Placement of a sling
    c. Dynamic splint
    d. Keeping the arm extended using pillow rolls

6. A patient being examined by the nurse has McBurney's point tenderness and a positive jar sign. Which of the following is the most likely diagnosis?
    a. Pyelonephritis
    b. Cholecystitis
    c. Appendicitis
    d. Meningitis

7. Which of the following triads describes signs of impending cerebral herniation?
    a. Beck's triad
    b. Charcot's triad
    c. Cushing's triad
    d. Bergman's triad

8. You are caring for a patient who received radiographic contrast medium for a procedure and the patient shows signs of dyspnea, flushing, and pruritis. Identify the top priority intervention:
    a. Check vital signs
    b. Ensure the airway is patent
    c. Apply a cold pack to the I.V. site
    d. Call the physician

9. According to Erikson's psychosocial model of development, which stage is typical of those who are elderly?
    a. Initiative vs. guilt
    b. Identity vs. role confusion
    c. Intimacy vs. isolation
    d. Ego integrity vs. despair

10. A patient with end stage renal carcinoma is found by the nurse to be making her funeral preparations. Which stage of Kübler-Ross's five stages of grief would best describe this patient?
    a. Anger
    b. Acceptance
    c. Bargaining
    d. Depression

11. According to Maslow's hierarchy, what is the second-highest level need required for survival and growth?
    a. Money
    b. Love
    c. Self-actualization
    d. Self esteem

12. What does the acronym OBRA stand for in regards to the care of nursing home residents?
    a. Office of Biomedical Research in America
    b. Oregon Biomedical Research Association
    c. Omnibus Budget Reconciliation Act
    d. Office of Budgeting and Research Association

13. A patient is being discharged from the hospital. During his hospital stay he was diagnosed with a deep vein thrombus in his right leg. Which of the following tests should be ordered as an outpatient to monitor this patient's condition?
    a. MRI
    b. CT scan
    c. Dopplers
    d. X-ray

14. A patient being examined by the nurse experiences pain when the nurse palpates her right upper quadrant with deep inspiration. What is this physical examination finding called?
    a. Psoas sign
    b. McBurney's sign
    c. Brudzinski sign
    d. Murphy's sign

15. You are giving Reglan to a patient with an ileus. The nursing student you are working with asks why Reglan is being given. Which of the following is the most appropriate response?
    a. "It stimulates gastric emptying."
    b. "It increases the rate of digestion."
    c. "It prevents diarrhea."
    d. "It treats acid reflux."

16. A patient is diagnosed with terminal lung cancer. Upon hearing the diagnosis, the patient blames his parents for smoking in his home when he was a child. Which stage of Kübler-Ross's five stages of grief would best describe this patient?
    a. Bargaining
    b. Depression
    c. Anger
    d. Denial

17. A patient is being evaluated for potential meningitis. Which of the following is NOT a typical sign/symptom associated with meningitis?
    a. Brudzinski sign
    b. Nystagmus
    c. Confusion
    d. Fever

18. A patient develops new-onset tremors on the right side of the body only. The patient remains awake and alert, although incredibly anxious, throughout the event until it spontaneously resolves. Which of the following is the most likely diagnosis?
    a. Grand mal seizure
    b. Tonic-clonic seizure
    c. Absence seizure
    d. Simple partial seizure

19. A patient admitted to the hospital after overdosing on Percocet should receive which of the following medications?
    a. Oxycodone
    b. Naloxone
    c. Prednisolone
    d. Flumazenil

20. A nurse is caring for a patient who has just begun to seize. Which of the following positions is the most appropriate for this patient to help prevent aspiration?
   a. Lateral recumbent
   b. Supine
   c. Trendelenburg
   d. Prone

21. Your hemodialysis patient has a positive 24-hour intake and output report. The physician plans to increase the frequency of treatment. Indicate the change you should suggest:
   a. Change the catheter
   b. Add heparin to the dialysate
   c. Increase the dialysate concentration
   d. Decrease the dialysate concentration

22. A patient with a subarachnoid hemorrhage is in moderate vasospasm. The family sees the nurse administering nimodipine to their family member and asks the nurse why she is doing so. Which of the following is the most appropriate response?
   a. "It is a beta blocker which causes the vessels to vasoconstrict."
   b. "It is a potassium channel blocker which causes the vessels to vasodilate."
   c. "It is a calcium channel blocker which causes the vessels to vasodilate."
   d. "It is a sodium channel blocker which causes the vessels to vasoconstrict."

23. What is the most common organism to cause epididymitis infections in the elderly or non–sexually active males?
   a. Cytomegalovirus
   b. *S. aureus*
   c. *N. Gonorrhea*
   d. *E. coli*

24. Your patient is in the oliguric phase of acute renal failure. Which physician order should you question?
   a. Administer sodium polystyrene sulfonate (Kayexalate)
   b. Limit oral fluids to 500 ml/24 hours
   c. Maintain a low-sodium, low-potassium, high-calorie diet
   d. Infuse IV fluids at 500 ml/hour

25. Identify the complication you would expect in a renal patient who had a large volume of fluid removed during hemodialysis:
   a. Leg and abdominal cramps
   b. Shortness of breath
   c. Chest pain
   d. Redness at the needle insertion site

26. You are caring for a patient receiving peritoneal dialysis, who continually remains in positive fluid balance. Choose the substance you would add to this patient's peritoneal dialysate to remove more fluid:
    a. Potassium
    b. Dextrose
    c. Urea
    d. Heparin

27. The nurse notices that a patient's hands and feet become erythematous when the patient is warm and pale, almost cyanotic, when the patient's hands and feet are uncovered. Which of the following is the most likely diagnosis?
    a. Turner syndrome
    b. Osgood-Schlatter disease
    c. Raynaud's disease
    d. Down syndrome

28. One hour after hemodialysis, your patient develops headache and confusion. Choose the complication you suspect:
    a. Hemorrhagic shock
    b. Dialysis disequilibrium syndrome
    c. Intracranial hemorrhage
    d. Hyperkalemia

29. While placing a Foley catheter in a female patient, a nurse notices a bluish discoloration of the vaginal mucosa. The patient is known to be pregnant. The name for this bluish discoloration is
    a. Levine sign.
    b. Kerning's sign.
    c. Chadwick sign.
    d. Obturator sign.

30. A patient suffers from a significant left middle cerebral artery stroke. The patient is right-handed. Which of the following deficits could the family expect to see in this patient?
    a. Left-sided weakness, visual deficits
    b. Right-sided weakness, visual deficits
    c. Right-sided weakness, speech deficits
    d. Left-sided weakness, speech deficits

31. Treatment of asymptomatic sinus bradycardia includes
    a. continuous telemetry monitoring.
    b. dopamine.
    c. epinephrine.
    d. vasopressin.

32. A patient is diagnosed with a lateral wall ST segment elevation myocardial infarction (STEMI). What do you expect the EKG to show?
    a. ST elevation in leads V1 – V6
    b. ST elevation in leads I, aVL, V5, V6
    c. ST elevation in leads II, III, aVF
    d. ST elevation in leads V7, V8, V9

33. Your type 1 diabetes mellitus patient is admitted with ketoacidosis. Choose the nursing diagnosis that takes top priority for this diabetic:
    a. Imbalanced nutrition: less than body requirements
    b. Deficient fluid volume
    c. Impaired tissue integrity
    d. Risk for infection

34. Your patient's diagnosis is adrenal crisis. Identify the electrolyte imbalance that is common with adrenal crisis:
    a. Hyperglycemia
    b. Hypernatremia
    c. Hypokalemia
    d. Hyponatremia

35. A patient develops diabetes insipidus after surgery to remove a pituitary tumor. Identify the critical complication of diabetes insipidus:
    a. Bradycardia
    b. Hyponatremia
    c. Dehydration
    d. Hypokalemia

36. A patient has metabolic alkalosis. Which of the following best describes that condition?
    a. HCO3 32, pH 7.50, CO2 37
    b. HCO3 26, pH 7.45, CO2 35
    c. HCO3 24, pH 7.35, CO2 40
    d. HCO3 19, pH 7.30, CO2 50

37. A patient undergoes gastrectomy for treatment of stomach cancer. Identify the complication most likely to develop following gastrectomy:
    a. Folic acid deficiency anemia
    b. Pernicious anemia
    c. Pancytopenia
    d. Thrombocytopenia

38. A patient develops a pruritic rash after being given an antibiotic and is given Benadryl for relief of her symptoms. The nurse should educate the patient about which of the following most common side effects?
    a. Cough
    b. Flushing
    c. Arthralgias
    d. Sedation

39. A patient who has developed cerebral edema is given Mannitol and Lasix. The nurse can expect which of the following changes in the patient's serum lab values?
    a. Increased sodium
    b. Increased platelet count
    c. Increased glucose
    d. Increased white blood cell count

40. You are teaching the parents of a child diagnosed with sickle cell disease about the disorder. Identify which instructions are appropriate for the parents:
    a. Apply cold to the affected areas to reduce the child's discomfort
    b. Restrict fluids during sickle cell crisis
    c. Avoid areas of low-oxygen concentration
    d. Exercise reduces the likelihood of crisis

41. When caring for a patient with pancreatitis, your first priority should be:
    a. Inserting an NG tube
    b. Inserting a urinary catheter
    c. Administering I.V. fluids and replacing electrolytes
    d. Encouraging oral fluid intake

42. Identify the circumstance in which a Living Will is appropriate:
    a. The patient is incapacitated and is terminally ill
    b. The patient is incapacitated and has a life-threatening but curable illness
    c. The patient was competent to express his wishes, desired treatment, and
       subsequently became incapacitated
    d. The patient is competent but wants his grown children to make health care decisions
       for him

43. A nurse is educating a patient with hyperthyroidism when the patient asks "What is the most common cause?" Which of the following is the most appropriate response?
    a. Hashimoto's disease
    b. Graves' disease
    c. Diabetes mellitus
    d. Addison's disease

44. Which of the following is NOT a complication of diabetes mellitus?
    a. Obesity
    b. Renal insufficiency
    c. Blindness
    d. Anemia

45. During which stage of the nurse-client relationship does the nurse assume different roles to help the patient cope?
    a. Fixation
    b. Orientation
    c. Exploration
    d. Termination

46. When giving Haldol, a nurse should educate the patient and family about which common side effect?
    a. Polyphagia
    b. Facial swelling
    c. Tardive dyskinesia
    d. Bradycardia

47. A 40-year-old female with no significant past medical history asks her nurse at what age should she undergo her first colonoscopy. She notes that her uncle died of colon cancer when he was 82. Which of the following is the most appropriate response?
 a. This year
 b. In 5 years
 c. In 10 years
 d. In 15 years

48. A patient was given Demerol for pain and has declining mental status and decreased respiratory rate. What medication can be given as an antidote for opiates?
 a. Mucomyst
 b. Naloxone
 c. Romazicon
 d. Activated charcoal

49. Which of the following patients are the least likely to be ordered Plavix?
 a. A patient with an ischemic stroke
 b. A patient with esophageal varices
 c. A patient who underwent a CABG
 d. A patient who recently suffered from an MI

50. Which of the following signs/symptoms are NOT caused by an atropine overdose?
 a. Hallucinations
 b. Blurred vision
 c. Diaphoresis
 d. Jaundice

51. Which of the following is the most common congenital cyanotic heart defect?
 a. Ventricular septal defect
 b. Tricuspid atresia
 c. Aortic stenosis
 d. Tetralogy of Fallot

52. Which of the following is NOT a complication in patients who have sickle cell anemia?
 a. Pulmonary embolus
 b. Myocardial infarction
 c. Esophageal varices
 d. Anemia

53. A male patient confides in his nurse about his sadness and anxiety after being diagnosed with a brain tumor. He denies hallucinations or suicidal ideation. Which of the following medications may help this patient?
 a. Haldol
 b. Keppra
 c. Lexapro
 d. Levoxyl

54. A patient's son becomes hysterical when he learns that his mother has suffered a massive stroke. He begins to yell obscenities at the nurse. Which of the following actions is the most appropriate for the nurse to take at this time?
   a. Call the police to arrest the patient's son for inappropriate behavior.
   b. Call the social worker to speak with the patient's son.
   c. Explain to the patient's son about the pathophysiology of a stroke.
   d. Educate the patient's son about Kübler-Ross's stages of grief.

55. A patient has just been diagnosed with diabetes insipidus. What is the drug of choice for treating this condition?
   a. Kayexalate
   b. Insulin
   c. Desmopressin
   d. Decadron

56. A patient admitted to the hospital is currently on a regimen of penicillin, which was started yesterday. Today the nurse notices diffuse rash and facial swelling. The patient states that he's never had this rash before. He has no drug allergies. He has no significant past medical history. On physical exam the nurse notices diffuse dark reddish purple papular rash on his trunk, face, and extremities with extensive blister formation. His temperature is 99.9; otherwise his vitals are normal. Based on his history and physical exam, what is the most likely diagnosis?
   a. Turner syndrome
   b. Steven-Johnson syndrome
   c. Cushing syndrome
   d. Guillain-Barré syndrome

57. A 25-year-old female is admitted to the hospital for fever of unknown origin. She has a temperature of 102.3 and is complaining of fever, chills, and diaphoresis. She has a known history of IV drug abuse. Your nursing student notes that the patient has Janeway lesions. Based on her history and physical exam, the most likely diagnosis is
   a. pneumonia.
   b. meningitis.
   c. endocarditis.
   d. *C. difficile* colitis.

58. Which of the following is a first-line treatment for Hashimoto's thyroiditis?
   a. Lantus
   b. Levothyroxine
   c. Tapazole
   d. Propylthiouracil

59. Which of the following is a treatment for active tuberculosis?
   a. Clindamycin
   b. Gentamicin
   c. Streptomycin
   d. Penicillin

60. A nurse is examining a patient who is in the hospital for acute asthma exacerbation. He has a known history of using nebulizers. During the physical exam, the nurse notices that he has cheesy white patches on his tongue that can be scraped off. This condition is called
    a. leukoplakia.
    b. oral thrush.
    c. parotitis.
    d. gingivostomatitis.

61. Which of the following would be a treatment of choice in an acute asthma exacerbation?
    a. Mucinex
    b. Xopenex
    c. Singulair
    d. Augmentin

62. Which of the following is a complication of paraphimosis?
    a. Mastitis
    b. Palpitations
    c. Cardiac arrhythmias
    d. Gangrene

63. A patient has just been diagnosed with glucose-6-phosphate dehydrogenase deficiency (G6PD deficiency). The parents ask the nurse which stimuli can cause outbreak of symptoms. Which of the following answers are most appropriate?
    a. Dairy products such as yogurt and ice cream
    b. Seafood, red meat, and alcohol
    c. Gluten-based products
    d. Sulfa drugs and aspirin

64. Which of the following is TRUE regarding sickle cell anemia?
    a. It is an autosomal dominant disease.
    b. Heterozygotes are usually asymptomatic.
    c. It is due to a defective chromosome 18.
    d. It increases your risk of diabetes.

65. A stroke patient in the ICU was supposed to receive a mechanical soft pureed diet due to her high risk of aspiration. The patient was accidentally ordered a regular diet by the medical team. When the patient ate her meal she aspirated and went into respiratory distress requiring intubation. While on the ventilator she developed pneumonia. Azithromycin was ordered for this patient. The patient had a documented allergy to macrolides, which was missed by the medical team. The patient developed anaphylaxis and died. How many sentinel events occurred during the patient's hospital stay?
    a. One
    b. Two
    c. Three
    d. Four

66. A patient with a subarachnoid hemorrhage is scheduled to receive Nimotop by mouth. The nurse in training accidentally gives the patient Nimotop IV and the patient's blood pressure drops to 50/20. The patient develops a small ischemic stroke following the event. How many sentinel events occurred during the patient's hospital stay?
    a. One
    b. Two
    c. Three
    d. Four

67. Which of the following is NOT a sign/symptom of hypoglycemia?
    a. Diaphoresis
    b. Altered mental status
    c. Fruity-smelling breath
    d. Palpitations

68. Which of the following is a sign/symptom of hypocalcemia?
    a. Nephrolithiasis
    b. Abdominal pain
    c. Chvostek's sign
    d. Bony pain

69. A 68-year-old man with a history of alcoholism has developed sudden onset of severe epigastric pain radiating to the back after eating. The pain is exacerbated when the patient lies flat or walks. He is pale and tachycardic and has nausea and vomiting and a temperature of 39° C. Physical examination shows the upper abdomen is tender but not rigid and without guarding. The most likely cause of these symptoms is:
    a. hepatitis
    b. acute cholecystitis
    c. small bowel obstruction
    d. pancreatitis

70. A patient has a permanent pacemaker. Which of the following scans are usually contraindicated in this patient?
    a. Ultrasound
    b. X-ray
    c. CT angiogram
    d. MRI

71. The medical team orders an EKG for a patient experiencing chest pain. The nurse attempts to apply the electrodes to the patient's chest, but his chest is incredibly hairy and the electrodes won't stick. Which of the following is the most appropriate action?
    a. Have the patient get a 2D echo instead.
    b. Forgo the EKG.
    c. Shave the patient's chest.
    d. Place electrodes on the back instead of on the chest.

72. A nurse is trying to obtain consent from an elderly patient who is hearing impaired. Which of the following actions is most inappropriate?
    a. Facing the patient while speaking
    b. Acting out the surgical procedure
    c. Speaking in a loud clear voice
    d. Having the patient read the consent themselves

73. Which of the following is NOT a treatment of ketoacidosis?
    a. Lantus
    b. IV fluids
    c. Kayexalate
    d. D50

74. While being interviewed, a patient tells her nurse that she develops anaphylaxis when exposed to IV contrast and seafood. Which of the following is contraindicated in this patient?
    a. Ultrasound
    b. CT angiogram
    c. MRI
    d. X-ray

75. You are caring for a 61-year-old female patient with known family history of hyperlipidemia. She has diabetes and high blood pressure which are controlled with medications. Which of the following is NOT a risk factor for coronary artery disease in this patient?
    a. Age
    b. Sex
    c. Diabetes
    d. Family history

76. A patient has developed anaphylaxis after she was given penicillin. She has remained conscious. Her vitals are pulse 122, BP 108/68, RR 38, O2 76% on non-rebreather (NRB) mask. She is also vomiting and has developed a diffuse body rash. Which of the following should be the initial step in stabilizing this patient?
    a. Intubate
    b. Administer Zofran
    c. Begin CPR
    d. Administer Benadryl

77. Which of the following is NOT a sign/symptom of anaphylaxis?
    a. Angioedema
    b. Urinary/bowel retention
    c. Cardiac arrest
    d. Respiratory distress

78. A pregnant patient is being given oxytocin by the medical team. As the nurse hangs the oxytocin infusion the patient asks the nurse why oxytocin is being given. What is the most appropriate response about oxytocin's primary function in this scenario?
    a. "It promotes and strengthens uterine contractions."
    b. "It helps alleviate pain."
    c. "It decreases the risk of newborn jaundice."
    d. "It prevents hemolytic disease of the newborn."

79. A nurse should wear which of the following when caring for a patient with *C. difficile* colitis?
    a. Gown and hair cap
    b. Hair cap, gloves, mask
    c. Mask, gown, gloves
    d. Gown, hair cap, and mask

80. A woman in the hospital has heavy menses, prolonged bleeding time, and chronic anemia. This patient should be screened for which of the following diseases?
    a. Turner syndrome
    b. Down syndrome
    c. Von Willebrand disease
    d. Parkinson's disease

81. A patient who is 24-hour postoperative after a pulmonary lobectomy requests pain medication for severe pain, but when the nurse brings the opioid medication a few minutes later, the nurse finds the patient laughing and talking with family. The nurse should
    a. give the patient the opioid medication.
    b. ask the patient if she still needs the pain medication.
    c. withhold the pain medication altogether.
    d. exchange the opioid for acetaminophen.

82. A 50-year-old bedridden patient has unilateral painful swelling of the lower extremity and a positive Homan's sign. This patient has no significant past medical history and no history of trauma. The leg is not erythematous or cyanotic. There are no palpable cords. Which of the following should be in the nurse's list of differential diagnoses?
    a. Compartment syndrome
    b. Raynaud's disease
    c. Deep vein thrombus
    d. Phlebitis

83. Which of the following is not a risk factor for developing listeriosis?
    a. Alcohol
    b. Raw vegetables
    c. Hot dogs
    d. Unpasteurized milk

84. A patient who is restless pulls out his chest tube when trying to get out of bed independently, and no dressing supplies are available at bedside. What immediate action is indicated?
   a. Call for assistance and dressing supplies.
   b. Hold a folded washcloth against the insertion site.
   c. Cover the insertion site with a clean, gloved hand.
   d. Ask the patient to place his hand over insertion site and go for dressings.

85. A patient with a history of heart failure and supraventricular dysrhythmias has been maintained on digoxin but has developed bradycardia (48 bpm), headache, fatigue, nausea, diarrhea, and green halo vision. The physician has ordered serum digoxin, electrolyte levels, and continuous ECG monitoring. Which of the following electrolyte values would be most concerning?
   a. Potassium of 3.2 mEq/L
   b. Potassium of 5 mEq/L
   c. Sodium 140 mEq/L
   d. Magnesium 2 mEq/L

86. A patient has been diagnosed with Parkinson's disease. The patient's family member asks the patient's nurse what causes Parkinson's disease. Which of the following is the most appropriate response?
   a. "It is caused the destruction of the substantia nigra which causes cognitive and motor deficits."
   b. "It is caused by the destruction of the basal ganglia which causes cognitive deficits."
   c. "It is caused by the destruction of muscle tissue which causes motor deficits."
   d. "It is caused by the destruction of the basal ganglia and muscle tissue which causes cognitive and motor deficits."

87. A patient has been diagnosed with Addison's disease. The patient's family member asks the patient's nurse what causes Addison's disease. Which of the following is the most appropriate response?
   a. "It is due to a lack of testosterone."
   b. "It is due to an excess of human growth hormone."
   c. "It is due to an excess of estrogen."
   d. "It is due to a lack of cortisol."

88. A patient's wife calls the ICU. She gives the required password to the patient's nurse to ensure her identity. She states that she will not be able to make it to the hospital today and wants to give consent for surgery over the phone. Which of the following is the most appropriate response?
   a. "You are not allowed to give consent over the phone. You have to be in the hospital to sign all consents."
   b. "You can give consent over the phone, but you will have to speak to a second nurse to witness that you are giving consent."
   c. "If you can't come to the hospital to sign consents, you should assign someone else to be power of attorney."
   d. "You can't give consent over the phone, but you can send another family member in your place to sign consents."

- 62 -

89. A 69-year-old male patient has persistent difficulty urinating. He complains of urinary frequency, but decreased urine output. His abdomen is distended and tender. His bladder scan shows a full bladder. His urinalysis is normal. Which of the following may provide relief?
    a. Dobbhoff
    b. Foley catheter
    c. Nasogastric tube
    d. Coude catheter

90. An agitated patient pulls his nasogastric tube (NGT) halfway out. The patient needs the NGT to receive tube feeds and medications. Several of his medications are due now. What is the most appropriate action to be taken by the nurse?
    a. Restart tube feeds and medications with the NGT in its current position.
    b. Advance the NGT to its prior position and restart tube feeds and medications.
    c. Pull the NGT out, reinsert another, and obtain a chest x-ray.
    d. Pull out the NGT and attempt to give oral medications and diet.

91. A patient who often gets kidney stones asks his nurse what he can do to prevent future recurrences. All of the following are appropriate responses except:
    a. decrease protein intake.
    b. decrease sodium intake.
    c. increase calcium intake.
    d. increase fluid intake.

92. Which of the following interventions is inappropriate for a non-infected Stage II decubitus ulcer?
    a. Wound care consult
    b. Surgical debridement
    c. Frequent repositioning
    d. Barrier cream

93. Which of the following medications is inappropriate for the treatment of Ménière's disease?
    a. Antivert
    b. Zofran
    c. Lasix
    d. Haloperidol

94. A 55-year-old patient with a known history of tobacco abuse and hypertension has not seen a doctor in over 10 years. He states that he feels fine. Secondary prevention in the patient would include
    a. colonoscopy.
    b. education regarding tobacco abuse.
    c. pneumococcal vaccine.
    d. physical examination.

95. A nurse is caring for a patient who has just returned from the operating room for an open cholecystectomy. The patient is vomiting and crying that she is in pain. The nurse notices a stage I decubitus ulcer on the patient's hip. The nurse also notices that one-third of the incision has opened up and is actively bleeding. Which of the following issues should be addressed first?
   a. Pain
   b. Nausea
   c. Incision
   d. Decubitus ulcer

96. Which of the following is NOT a Joint Commission national patient safety goal?
   a. Identify patients that are at high risk for suicide.
   b. Use at least one form of identification before giving medication.
   c. Follow Centers for Disease Control (CDC) hand cleaning guidelines.
   d. Relay important test/lab results to the correct person in a timely manner.

97. A nursing student and his preceptor are evaluating their patients at the start of their day shift. They are caring for a psychiatric patient complaining of chest pain with stable vital signs, a patient status post open appendectomy yesterday who is currently sleeping, a patient with a subdural hematoma complaining of headache who is more lethargic, and a patient with a femur fracture requesting more pain medication. Which of these patients should be seen last?
   a. Patient with the subdural hematoma
   b. Patient with the femur fracture
   c. Patient complaining of chest pain
   d. Patient status post appendectomy

98. A nurse receives a phone call from the lab stating that a patient's serum potassium is 6.5 but it is hemolyzed. Which of the following is the most appropriate step in intervention?
   a. Send repeat serum potassium now.
   b. Send the patient for a 2D echo.
   c. Send a troponin level and administer baby aspirin.
   d. No intervention

99. A nurse accidentally splashes himself in the eye with a chemical solution. All of the following are appropriate actions except
   a. going to Employee Health and reporting the incident.
   b. calling his nurse manager.
   c. placing an eye patch over the affected eye and continuing to work.
   d. irrigating the eye with water flushes.

100. A nurse caring for a patient with a chest tube notices continuous bubbling in the water-seal chamber. The nurse has determined that the leak is inside of the chest. Which of the following is the most appropriate intervention?
   a. Place the chest tube on suction until the air leak resolves.
   b. Clamp the tubing indefinitely.
   c. No intervention
   d. Pull out the chest tube.

101. A patient has just undergone a surgical abortion. A male calls the surgery center and identifies himself as the patient's husband. He asks the patient's nurse what kind of procedure the patient had. Which of the following is the most appropriate response?

    a. "That's not your business."
    b. "If you give me your name and phone number I can have the patient call you back."
    c. "The patient had a surgical abortion and did not have any intraoperative or postoperative complications."
    d. "The patient had an abortion, but I am not allowed to tell you which type or if any complications occurred."

102. Which of the following measures will NOT help alleviate headache status post lumbar puncture?

    a. Tylenol
    b. Reverse Trendelenburg
    c. Epidural blood patch
    d. Rest

103. A patient is admitted for hypertensive crisis. He states that he is on four antihypertensive medications, but is not compliant with any of them because it's difficult to remember when to take them. Which of the following is the most appropriate response by the nurse?

    a. "It's not that hard to remember to take medications."
    b. "If you don't start taking medications you will die from renal, cardiac, or neurological complications."
    c. "While it may be difficult to remember all of them, even if you take one or two medications it would help your blood pressure."
    d. "If it's difficult for you to remember to take all of your medications, why don't you set an alarm that goes off every time a pill is due?"

104. With chronic kidney disease, potassium-sparing diuretics are recommended for

    a.   patients with persistent hypokalemia.
    b.   all patients with chronic kidney disease.
    c.   patients with hyporeninemic hypoaldosteronism.
    d.   patients who cannot tolerate hydrochlorothiazide.

105. Which of the following reflects a tertiary intervention?

    a. Ordering a mammogram for a patient with a family history of breast cancer
    b. Educating a patient about the importance of physical activity
    c. Undergoing a diverting colostomy for a stage III decubitus ulcer of the buttock
    d. Administering a vaccine to adolescent females to prevent cervical cancer

106. A patient being treated for acute alcohol intoxication has a banana bag being infused. The patient's family member asks the nurse why the patient needs a banana bag. Which of the following is NOT a correct response?

    a. "It prevents the occurrence of a hangover."
    b. "It helps to rehydrate the patient."
    c. "It helps to correct electrolyte abnormalities."
    d. "It provides the patient with vitamins that she may be deficient in after drinking alcohol."

107. A patient is being given Synthroid. The patient's family member asks the nurse why the patient is being given this medication. What is the most appropriate response?
    a. "It acts as a synthetic thyroid hormone to treat the patient's hyperthyroidism."
    b. "It acts as synthetic insulin to treat the patient's diabetes."
    c. "It acts as a synthetic thyroid hormone to treat the patient's hypothyroidism."
    d. "It acts as synthetic growth hormone to treat the patient's dwarfism."

108. A 72-year-old man underwent a total knee replacement. Prior to surgery he was alert, responsive, and oriented, but 24 hours after surgery he is having fluctuating periods of confusion with sudden changes in consciousness, inability to sustain attention, disorientation, and visual hallucinations. The most effective pharmaceutical intervention is
    a. lorazepam (Ativan).
    b. benztropine (Cogentin).
    c. chlordiazepoxide (Librium).
    d. paroxetine (Paxil).

109. A patient with stress incontinence asks her nurse if there's anything she can do to help alleviate symptoms. Which of the following is NOT an appropriate suggestion?
    a. Take frequent bathroom breaks.
    b. Practice Kegel exercises.
    c. Avoid/limit alcohol.
    d. Increase caffeine intake.

110. A patient who has suffered a serious stroke has problems toileting and dressing himself independently. He is scheduled to be discharged in two days. Which of the following is NOT an appropriate action to be taken by the nurse?
    a. Tell the patient he has to go to a nursing home upon discharge.
    b. Talk to the social worker about setting up a home health aide.
    c. Educate the patient's wife on how to assist her husband at home.
    d. Talk to the medical team about the possible need for rehab.

111. A patient's family has just discovered that their loved one's traumatic brain injury is a life-ending injury, and comfort measures only (CMO) is recommended by the attending physician. While the nurse is in the room repositioning the patient, the family is crying and yelling obscenities. Which of the following actions is NOT an appropriate action to be taken by the nurse at this time?
    a. Ask them to lower their voices or go to a private family room.
    b. Close the door to give the patient's family privacy.
    c. Ask the patient's family if they would like a religious leader called.
    d. Ask the family if the patient wanted her organs donated.

112. Which of the following is NOT a treatment for a patient with ineffective airway clearance but patent airway?
    a. Insert an LMA.
    b. Perform chest percussion.
    c. Administer medications that reduce secretions.
    d. Encourage use of the incentive spirometer.

113. An elderly female patient was brought to the ER for altered mental status and has now been admitted to a medical surgical unit. She lives in a basement apartment with family, but the family can't remember the last time they saw her at her neurological baseline. They admit to not seeing her for six days. She is covered in new and old excrement, has multiple ecchymoses, and has two decubitus ulcers. After attending to the immediate medical needs of the patient, which is the most appropriate nursing intervention?
    a. Interview each of the family members individually.
    b. Contact the hospital social worker.
    c. Recommend an assisted nursing facility to the family.
    d. Take pictures of the wounds and send them to the police.

114. Which of the following reflects a primary intervention?
    a. Receiving a tetanus shot as a routine immunization
    b. Undergoing a routine colonoscopy
    c. Undergoing a mastectomy for breast cancer
    d. Placing a chest tube for a pneumothorax

115. A patient has stepped on a rusty nail. Her last tetanus shot was five years ago. When should she receive another tetanus shot?
    a. Now
    b. One year
    c. Five years
    d. Ten years

116. A patient is admitted for suspected malaria. Family members ask the nurse how their loved one got this disease. Which of the following is the most appropriate answer?
    a. "It was transmitted by an infected mosquito."
    b. "It is a sexually transmitted disease."
    c. "It is transmitted by ticks."
    d. "It is a highly aggressive cancer."

117. A patient with a tracheostomy is to receive the Passy-Muir valve to facilitate communication and improve swallowing. What change must be made when placing the valve on the tracheostomy tube?
    a.   Cuff deflated
    b.   Cuff inflation increased
    c.   No changes necessary
    d.   Cuff inflation decreased by approximately 50%.

118. What is the treatment for syphilis in its early stages?
    a. No intervention
    b. Diflucan
    c. Miconazole cream
    d. Penicillin

119. A patient who is taking metformin for diabetes mellitus, type 2, is also taking metoprolol for junctional tachycardia and has been prescribed hydrochlorothiazide for persistent elevated blood pressure. What is the primary concern with this drug combination?
   a. Increased tachycardia
   b. Hyperglycemia
   c. Renal failure
   d. Muscle cramps

120. A patient has recently been diagnosed with celiac disease after tests to determine the cause of chronic weight loss, anemia, diarrhea, rash, bone pain, and irregular menses. When discussing dietary interventions, the nurse tells the patient that celiac disease may result in malabsorption of
   a. vitamin B_{12}.
   b. folate and iron.
   c. vitamin C.
   d. vitamin D.

121. A patient who is CMO (Comfort Measures Only) currently has a blood pressure of 68/30. Which of the following is the most appropriate intervention?
   a. Administer a fluid bolus.
   b. No intervention.
   c. Call the attending physician.
   d. Start a vasopressor infusion.

122. A nurse is coming on for his day shift and enters a patient's room. The night shift nurse reported to him that there were no significant events during her shift. The patient is covered in excrement and urine, which seems to have been there for some time. Which of the following is the most appropriate action to be taken by the day nurse initially?
   a. Clean the patient and attend to his needs.
   b. Call the nursing manager.
   c. Schedule a confliction resolution meeting with the night nurse.
   d. Call the night nurse at home and reprimand her.

123. A 56-year-old female oncology arrives on the unit as a direct admit. As she is being assisted to her bed from the wheelchair, she is noted to have extreme shortness of breath. She is found to be hypoxic, but her vitals are otherwise stable. Which of the following is the most appropriate action to be taken by the nurse initially?
   a. Begin preparations for chest tube placement.
   b. Perform a history and physical.
   c. Perform an EKG.
   d. Place the patient on a non-rebreather (NRB) mask.

124. Which of the following changes in fluid intelligence are associated with age?
   a. Decreased test anxiety
   b. Altered time perception
   c. Decreased long-term memory
   d. Increased reaction time

- 68 -

125. A night nurse is signing out to the day nurse during change of shift. They are assessing a patient with a traumatic head injury who, per the night nurse, was neurologically intact one hour ago and is now lethargic and confused. Which of the following is the most appropriate action to be taken by the nurses?

    a. The day nurse should re-evaluate the exam in one hour.

    b. The night nurse should change her documentation overnight to reflect the new exam findings.

    c. One or both nurses should call the attending physician.

    d. The day nurse should report the night nurse to the nurse manager for incompetence.

126. A patient diagnosed with a stroke received tissue plasminogen activator (tPA) five hours ago and now has urinary incontinence. The patient has moderate motor deficits, but she remains cognizant. Which of the following is the most appropriate nursing intervention for this patient?

    a. Offer the patient a bed pan often.

    b. Call a nephrology consult.

    c. Place a Foley.

    d. Have the patient ambulate to the commode.

127. A patient is being discharged on Keppra and asks her nurse the purpose of this medication. What is the most appropriate response?

    a. "It prevents deep vein thromboses."

    b. "It improves high blood pressure."

    c. "It prevents and treats seizures."

    d. "It softens bowel movements."

128. A patient's blood pressure is 95/55 and the patient is resting comfortably in bed. The patient is scheduled to receive Norvasc. The nurse looks back to the original order, but no parameters were written. Which of the following is the most appropriate nursing intervention?

    a. Hold the Norvasc for now.

    b. Give double the dose of Norvasc.

    c. Give the Norvasc as scheduled.

    d. Call the attending and clarify parameters.

129. A patient whose intermittent claudication had progressed to rest pain and had not responded to conservative treatment has undergone a fem-pop bypass. The patient complains of numbness and tingling on the anterior and medial aspect of the leg. This suggests

    a.   damage to the femoral nerve.

    b.   occlusion of the femoral artery.

    c.   normal postoperative sensation.

    d.   bypass occlusion.

130. A nurse coming on for her day shift is assigned to care for a patient with an acute myocardial infarction who is currently asymptomatic, a patient status post cholecystectomy who is sleeping, a patient with a brain tumor scheduled to go to the operating room this morning, and a patient with pancreatitis who is scheduled to go home today. Which of the following patients should the nurse see first?
   a. The patient with the myocardial infarction
   b. The patient with pancreatitis
   c. The patient with the brain tumor
   d. The patient status post cholecystectomy

131. Which of the following is the most likely day for a fever to occur due to a wound infection in a post-operative patient?
   a. POD 1
   b. POD 5
   c. POD 10
   d. POD 15

132. A patient has had the following blood sugar levels over the past 12 hours: 266, 354, 275, and 401. The patient has a known history of diabetes. Which of the following is NOT an appropriate nursing intervention?
   a. Request to increase the patient's sliding scale insulin.
   b. Request to change the patient from regular diet to a diabetic diet.
   c. Tell the patient he needs to ask the attending to consult an endocrinologist.
   d. Educate the patient about the risks of uncontrolled diabetes.

133. A nurse is taking care of a patient who has just been admitted for a hemorrhagic stroke. The patient's blood pressure is 201/112. The patient's neurological exam is stable. The patient's blood sugar is 75. The patient is vomiting. While doing an examination the ICU nurse notes that the patient is covered in feces. Which of the following should the nurse address first?
   a. Cleaning the patient
   b. The patient's nausea
   c. The patient's blood sugar
   d. The patient's blood pressure

134. Which of the following drugs puts the patient with diabetes mellitus, type 2, most at risk for episodes of acute hypoglycemia?
A. Metformin (Glucophage)
B. Rosiglitazone (Avandia)
C. Exenatide (Byetta)
D. Glipizide (Glucotrol)

135. A patient with a Foley catheter with normal renal function and previously normal urine output has had no urine output for several hours. The patient has no discomfort and her abdomen is not distended. Which of the following is the most appropriate initial intervention?
   a. Flush the Foley.
   b. Discontinue the Foley.
   c. Call the attending.
   d. Call a nephrology consult.

136. Which of the following is NOT contraindicated in a patient who has just received tissue plasminogen activator (tPA)?
    a. Foley catheter
    b. Central line
    c. Nasogastric tube
    d. Texas catheter

137. Which of the following is the most likely day for a fever to occur due to atelectasis in a post-operative patient?
    a. POD 1
    b. POD 3
    c. POD 5
    d. POD 7

138. A patient has been hospitalized with nausea and vomiting but minimal abdominal distention. The patient has not passed flatus in 14 hours, and abdominal x-ray shows dilated small bowel loops and no colonic or rectal gas. The patient's CBC and electrolytes are within normal limits. Based on these findings, the nurse should suspect that the primary initial intervention will be
    a.   contrast studies.
    b.   NG suction.
    c.   exploratory surgery.
    d.   observation.

139. A patient is experiencing delirium tremens. Which of the following is NOT an appropriate intervention?
    a. Administer Ativan.
    b. Keep the patient NPO.
    c. Administer a banana bag.
    d. Administer Reglan.

140. A patient receiving maintenance lithium at 300 mg three times daily for bipolar disorder has developed vomiting, diarrhea, tinnitus, and tremors. The patient's blood level is 1.8 mEq/L. The initial response should be to
    a.   withhold lithium.
    b.   increase lithium dosage.
    c.   decrease lithium dosage.
    d.   maintain lithium dosage and provide an antipsychotic medication.

141. A nurse coming on for his night shift is assigned to care for a patient with pneumonia who is sleeping, a patient with sepsis who just became lethargic, a patient with a subdural hematoma (SDH) scheduled to go to the OR tomorrow, and a patient with pancreatitis due to alcohol abuse who is going through withdrawal. Which one of his patients should be seen LAST?
    a. The septic patient
    b. The patient with pneumonia
    c. The patient with pancreatitis
    d. The patient with the SDH

142. Which of the following is the most likely day for a fever to occur due to a UTI in a post-operative patient?
    a. POD 1
    b. POD 3
    c. POD 7
    d. POD 10

143. A patient is being discharged with Lopressor. Which of the following is a common side effect that the nurse should educate the patient about?
    a. Angioedema
    b. Bruising
    c. Fatigue
    d. Flushing

144. A patient with sickle cell crisis has just been admitted to the unit. His oxygen saturation is 98% on nasal cannula. The patient is complaining of chest and extremity pain. The patient is vomiting. The patient's blood pressure is 92/58. Which one of the following issues can be addressed last?
    a. Pain
    b. Blood pressure
    c. Oxygen
    d. Nausea

145. A nurse arriving to the hospital for his day shift is caring for a patient who had an open cholecystectomy three days ago. The patient still has the original post-operative dressing. The previous nursing staff have documented that the incision site is clean and dry. What is the most appropriate initial action?
    a. Remove the dressing and check the incision.
    b. Call the nurse manager to report the incident.
    c. Leave the dressing on and sign it out to the night nurse.
    d. Document that the incision is clean and dry.

146. Which of the following is NOT an intervention to treat a patient with sickle cell crisis?
    a. Supplemental oxygen
    b. Narcotic pain medications
    c. IV fluids
    d. Cooling blankets

147. The nurse is reviewing preoperative laboratory values. The nurse should alert the physician to which of the following values?
    a. Glucose level of 98 mg/dL
    b. Blood, urea, nitrogen (BUN) level of 26 mg/dL
    c. Creatinine level of 0.79 mg/dL
    d. Calcium level of 0.2 mg/dL

148. A patient is being discharged on niacin. Which of the following is a common side effect that the nurse should educate the patient about?
    a. Orange urine
    b. Cough
    c. Flushing
    d. Weight gain

149. Which of the following is the most likely day for a drug fever to occur in a post-operative patient?
    a. POD 1
    b. POD 3
    c. POD 5
    d. POD 7

150. A 25-year-old patient is being discharged after undergoing a repair of a cerebral aneurysm. Prior to admission the patient had had no pertinent medical problems or family history and has had a healthy lifestyle. Which of the following is the most important thing to tell the family members?
    a. "Immediate family members should be screened for aneurysms."
    b. "Cigarette smoking plays a large role in the development of aneurysms."
    c. "This was an isolated event and family members shouldn't be concerned."
    d. "Aneurysms are more common in younger patients."

Answers and Explanations

1. A: Food, water, sleep, and excretion are the four fundamental needs according to Maslow's hierarchy. These needs have to be fulfilled in order for a person to have a sense of peace and safety. The next level includes security of oneself and the safety of loved ones. The next level includes fulfillment of relationships with family members, friends, and intimacy with loved ones. Self-esteem is the second-highest level, followed by the highest level of self-actualization.

2. A: Monitor the patient for fluid and electrolyte imbalances
Ileostomy drainage contains large amounts of fluid and electrolytes from the upper GI tract. Hence, monitoring the patient's fluid and electrolyte status is crucial to prevent dehydration. Proteolytic enzymes are used for patients with pancreatic failure. Ileostomies are never irrigated; instead, they have a continuous liquid drainage. Antidiarrheal medications are ineffective for the upper GI tract.

3. D: Give the medications that will be retained, and hold those that would be dialyzed out
Some medications may be dialyzed out of the blood with peritoneal dialysis or hemodialysis. Find out which of the patient's medications are affected by dialysis. If you cannot find a chart with this information, phone the pharmacist. Drugs that are not dialyzed out may be given. Hold drugs that are dialyzed out until after dialysis.

4. B: Administer I.V. fluid boluses, as prescribed
Prerenal failure is caused by decreased blood flow to the kidneys, which can lead to ischemia in the nephrons. I.V. fluid boluses may improve flow and improve perfusion to the nephrons. Antibiotics, oral hygiene, and repositioning are not priorities in this situation.

5. B: Placement of a sling will only worsen the contracture. The goal of prevention/treatment of contractures is to increase range of motion through exercises and by positioning. Surgery may also be used, but even after surgical correction the contracture may reoccur.

6. C: The diagnosis of acute appendicitis can sometimes be aided by physical examination findings. McBurney's point is found in the right lower quadrant two-thirds of the way between the navel and the anterior superior iliac spine. The jar sign is elicited when patients experience pain after they stand on their toes and drop to the soles of their feet. Pain is due to the jarring of the inflamed peritoneum caused by acute appendicitis. Neither of these signs are positive in the other test choices.

7. C: Cushing's triad is a clinical triad defined as hypertension, bradycardia, and irregular respirations. It suggests rising intracranial pressure due to intracranial pathology such as hemorrhage. Beck's triad is the combination of distended jugular veins, hypotension, and muffled heart sounds. It occurs as a result of pericardial effusion. Charcot's triad is the combination of jaundice, fever, and right upper quadrant abdominal pain. It occurs as a result of ascending cholangitis. Bergman's triad is the combination of dyspnea, petechiae, and mental status changes. It occurs when a patient has a fat embolism.

8. B: Ensure the airway is patent. The patient shows signs of an allergy to the iodine in the contrast medium. The first action is to ensure the patient's airway is patent. If the airway is compromised, call a cardiac arrest (Code Blue). Checking vital signs and calling for the physician are important nursing actions but should follow ensuring patency of the airway. A cold pack is not indicated.

9. D: Ego integrity versus despair is the last stage of Erikson's psychosocial theory of development. It occurs around the age of retirement (mid-sixties) and lasts until the end of a person's life. Those who have few regrets regarding their life choices and who are proud of their achievements and of their family will maintain their dignity and integrity until their death. Those who have made poor life choices or who doubt their life choices will become depressed, fearful, and bitter.

10. B: This patient has accepted the inevitability of her death and is making plans to help herself face it. The five stages include denial, anger, bargaining, depression, and acceptance. Not all people go through all of the stages of grief, nor are they necessarily experienced in a particular order. In some cases, patients return to one or more stages several times until they are able to work through it.

11. D: Food, water, sleep, and excretion are the four fundamental needs according to Maslow's hierarchy. These needs have to be fulfilled in order for a person to have a sense of peace and safety. The next level includes security of oneself and the safety of loved ones. The next level includes fulfillment of relationships with family members, friends, and intimacy with loved ones. Self-esteem is the second-highest level, followed by the highest level of self-actualization.

12. C: The Omnibus Budget Reconciliation Act (OBRA), also known as the Nursing Home Reform Act of 1987, mandates the minimum standards of care for nursing home facilities. These mandates cover aspects of care such as addressing each resident's medical, social, and emotional needs; preventing the decline of the ability to perform basic activities of daily life and providing assistance if those abilities do decline; incorporating safety measures; and other standards that keep nursing home residents reasonably healthy and comfortable.

13. C: Ultrasound Dopplers are the gold standard for diagnosing superficial vein thromboses (SVTs) and deep vein thromboses (DVTs). Not all patients are candidates to get MRIs (e.g., those with pacemakers or implantable metal devices). CT scans and MRIs are quite expensive and give off significantly more radiation than an ultrasound, which involves minimal radiation. These tests would not give any more information than an ultrasound could obtain; therefore, an ultrasound is preferable. X-rays only evaluate bones, so they are not useful when trying to evaluate the interior of a blood vessel.

14. D: A positive Murphy's sign aids in the diagnosis of acute cholecystitis. The psoas sign is positive if patients experience abdominal pain when they actively flex their leg at the hip and knee. This maneuver is used to help diagnose appendicitis. McBurney's sign is positive when patients have tenderness over McBurney's point. This point is found in the right lower quadrant two-thirds of the way between the navel and the anterior superior iliac spine. It is used to help diagnose appendicitis. The Brudzinski sign is positive when flexion of the neck usually causes flexion of the hip and knee. This maneuver is used to help diagnose meningitis.

15. A: An ileus is the loss of peristalsis of the GI tract caused by disease, spinal cord injury, or following recent surgery. Symptoms include constipation, abdominal distention, nausea, and vomiting. Decompression with a nasogastric tube is usually the first choice of initial treatment. Additional relief can be given by administering Reglan, which helps alleviate nausea and promotes gastric emptying.

16. C: This patient is in the anger phase. He blames his parents for his diagnosis instead of focusing on what he can do to face and prepare for his death. The five stages include denial, anger, bargaining, depression, and acceptance. Not all people go through all of the stages of grief, nor are they necessarily experienced in a particular order. In some cases, patients return to one or more stages several times until they are able to work through it.

17. B: Nystagmus is not a common finding in those afflicted with meningitis, although there are a few who may have it as one of their presenting symptoms. The classic triad of symptoms for meningitis is fever, altered mental status, and nuchal rigidity. The Brudzinski sign is positive when flexion of the neck usually causes flexion of the hip and knee. This maneuver is used to help diagnose meningitis.

18. D: A simple partial seizure presents with unilateral or generalized tremors, but the patient remains awake and alert throughout the entire seizure. Tonic-clonic seizures, also known as grand mal seizures, present with generalized body tremors, tongue biting, diaphoresis, and/or urinary or bowel incontinence followed by a postictal period. The patient usually has no memory of the seizure itself. Absence seizures are more common in children than adults. They can sometimes be misdiagnosed due to the unusual presentation of intermittent blank staring episodes.

19. B: Naloxone, also known as Narcan, is an opiate antidote to treat potential or confirmed narcotic overdoses. Prednisolone is a corticosteroid drug. It is useful for the treatment of a wide range of inflammatory and auto-immune conditions. Flumazenil, also known as Romazicon, is the antidote for benzodiazepines. Oxycodone is an opiate. All opiates can potentially cause sedation and should never be given to a lethargic patient or to someone who has a suspected opiate overdose.

20. A: The lateral recumbent position involves placing a patient on his side with the legs extended. This position helps prevent aspiration. A patient who is placed in the other positions has an increased risk of aspiration. When a patient is vomiting, seizing, or has respiratory distress, he should be sat up, placed on his side, or placed in reverse Trendelenburg to help ensure that his airway remains open and unobstructed.

21. C: The nurse should recommend increasing the dialysate concentration to address the positive intake and output report for this patient. Fluid moves from an area of lower particle concentration to an area of higher particle concentration. Dialysate with a higher concentration pulls more fluid across a semipermeable membrane, therefore dialysate with a higher concentration increases fluid removal. An increase in output is required to equalize the intake and output for this patient. The opposite occurs with a less concentrated dialysate and would only further increase the positive fluid balance in the patient. Heparin prevents clotting but does not improve fluid removal. The dialysis catheter should be changed only if it is obstructed. Providing fluid is draining without difficulty, the catheter is patent.

22. C: Nimodipine or Nimotop is a calcium channel blocker which causes vasodilation of the blood vessels. This is important when treating a patient with a subarachnoid hemorrhage in vasospasm. The "triple H" therapy for subarachnoid hemorrhage–induced vasospasm is hypervolemia, hypertension, and hemodilution. These three factors will maintain the patency of the vessels, making it difficult for them to vasoconstrict. Vasospasm left unchecked can cause stroke, neurological compromise, and death.

23. D: Epididymitis is commonly caused by *E.coli* in elderly males and/or those who are not sexually active and have normal immune function. In sexually active males with a history of unprotected sex, the causative organisms are likely gonorrhea and/or chlamydia. Cases of epididymitis caused by *Staph aureus* are rare. Epididymitis caused by cytomegalovirus (CMV) is incredibly rare unless the patient is immunocompromised.

24. D: The nurse should question the order to infuse IV fluids at 500 mL/hour during the oliguric phase of acute renal failure, due to its risk for causing fluid overload. During this phase, damage to the kidneys causes a drastic decrease in urine output, as low as 100-400mL/day. This increases the risk for hypervolemia (fluid overload), electrolyte imbalances and acidosis. Fluid restriction is a critical intervention in this stage of renal failure to prevent hypervolemia, therefore infusing IV fluids at 500mL/hour is inappropriate. Limiting oral fluids to 500mL/24 hours is an appropriate intervention for managing fluid balance. Administering sodium polystyrene sulfonate (Kayexalate) is used during this phase to lower serum potassium levels, and maintaining a low-sodium, low-potassium and high calorie diet also address the risk for electrolyte imbalances and nutrient needs during the oliguric phase.

25. A: Leg and abdominal cramps. A patient who has a large volume of fluid removed during hemodialysis can experience leg and abdominal cramping due to electrolyte loss. Fluid removal should make breathing easier, not cause shortness of breath. Chest pain is associated with excessive fluid gain. Redness at the insertion site may be a sign of infection and is not associated with fluid volume removed during hemodialysis.

26. B: Dextrose. Increasing the amount of dextrose in the peritoneal dialysate increases the osmotic gradient and draws additional water across the peritoneal dialyzing membrane. Potassium and heparin are occasionally added to dialysate, but they do not increase the amount of water removed. Urea is an osmotic agent at times, but is basically a waste product in the blood that is removed by dialysis.

27. C: Raynaud's disease is caused by the body's abnormal response to cold weather and to stress. The body significantly decreases the blood flow to the extremities, causing pallor or cyanosis and paresthesias in response to cold weather. A way to prevent or limit the severity of an exacerbation is to avoid cold exposure as much as possible by dressing in warm layers.

28. B: Dialysis disequilibrium syndrome. Rapid removal of urea from the blood favors osmotic movement of water toward the brain, where urea concentrations are initially higher. This can cause dialysis disequilibrium syndrome, which leads to confusion and headaches. There are no indications that the patient is experiencing blood loss. Intracranial hemorrhage would probably cause local neurologic deficits. Hyperkalemia should be resolved by dialysis.

29. C: In early pregnancy, high levels of estrogen cause increased venous pressure causing the mucosal surfaces of the genitals to turn a purplish or bluish color. The obturator sign is positive when abdominal pain is elicited with the internal rotation of the flexed right leg. This maneuver helps diagnose appendicitis. The Levine sign is positive when a patient is holding a clenched fist over his chest to describe dull, pressing chest pain consistent with the discomfort of angina pectoris. Kerning's sign is positive when a patient is unable to extend his leg when his hip is flexed. This maneuver helps diagnose meningitis.

30. C: The patient, like the majority of the population, is right-handed which means that she uses the left side of the brain predominantly. Since the brain controls the contralateral aspect of the body, a left-sided stroke would result in right-sided weakness. The middle cerebral territory is where most of the language centers of the brain are located. A significant MCA stroke would likely result in some degree of speech deficit. Visual deficits are usually caused by occipital lobe strokes.

31. A: Asymptomatic bradycardia requires monitoring, but no intervention. Symptoms of bradycardia may include pallor, weakness, dizziness, altered mental status, fatigue, and shortness of breath. If the patient had been symptomatic, atropine is the first-line agent used. In the event that atropine is ineffective, epinephrine and dopamine may be used. If patients display signs of poor perfusion, they may be candidates for transcutaneous pacing.

32. B: Choice B would show a lateral wall MI. Severe ischemia can result in EKG changes within minutes of the occurrence. Other helpful diagnostic aids would include troponin level, CK-MB level, and a 2D echo. These aids can be more diagnostic than an EKG, but an EKG result is obtained much quicker than blood work or a 2D echo. It takes a minimum of three hours for a cardiac insult to be reflected in blood tests. Choice A would show an anterior MI. Choice C would show an inferior wall MI. Choice D would show a posterior wall MI.

33. B: Deficient fluid volume In diabetic ketoacidosis, a severe disturbance in protein, fat, and carbohydrate metabolism results from profound insulin deficiency. Levels of counter-regulatory hormones (glucagon, cortisol, and growth hormone) are markedly increased and antagonize the effects of insulin. The patient develops severe hyperglycemia, osmotic diuresis, dehydration, hyperlipidemia, and metabolic acidosis. Electrolyte depletion occurs as ketones are lost in the urine. Osmotic diuresis leads to severe dehydration. Therefore, the priority nursing diagnosis is deficient fluid volume. The patient may need 4 to 6 L (3.8 to 5.7 qt) or more of normal saline for initial fluid replacement. Dehydration may lead to thirst, dry mucous membranes, skin turgor loss, renal failure, and hypovolemic shock. The other options are inappropriate in this case.

34. D: Hyponatremia. One key change in adrenal crisis is deficiency in the hormone aldosterone, a mineralocorticoid. Aldosterone regulates the reabsorption of sodium and the excretion of potassium by the kidneys. Deficiency of aldosterone leads to decreased sodium reabsorption in the distal tubules of the kidneys and increased sodium retention. Consequently, large amounts of sodium, chloride, and water are excreted in the urine, resulting in hyponatremia and depletion of extracellular fluid volume, hyperkalemia, and mild metabolic alkalosis. The patient in adrenal crisis will have hypoglycemia, not hyperglycemia.

35. D: Hypokalemia. The most dangerous complication for the patient is hypokalemia, caused by excessive diuresis. Low potassium levels can lead to cardiac arrhythmias, such as heart block, ventricular tachycardia, and cardiac arrest. Diabetes insipidus is associated with tachycardia and hypotension. The patient's serum sodium levels increase, because the body retains sodium as potassium is excreted. Dehydration is a complication, but is less serious than hypokalemia.

36. A: To interpret an arterial blood gas, first look at the pH. If it is low, acidosis is present. If the pH is high, alkalosis is present. A normal pH range is 7.35–7.45. Next look at $paCO_2$; if it is low, acidosis is present. If it is increased, alkalosis is present. The normal paCO2 range is 35–45. If the PaCO2 explains the change of pH, then it is a respiratory disorder. If not, look at the HCO3. The normal range is 22–26. If the HCO3 is increased and the pH is high, then you have metabolic alkalosis. If the pH is low and the HCO3 is low, you have metabolic acidosis.

37. B: Pernicious anemia. A gastrectomy removes the source of intrinsic factor, the stomach lining, which is needed to absorb Vitamin B12;. Folic acid is absorbed in the ileum and is unaffected by gastrectomy. Pancytopenia is depression of all cellular elements of the blood, and thrombocytopenia is decreased platelets. Neither of these hematological conditions is caused by gastrectomy.

38. D: Sedation is one of the most common side effects of Benadryl. It should never be given to a patient who will be driving, who has acute alcohol intoxication, or who is about to imbibe alcoholic beverages. A persistent idiopathic cough is a common side effect in ACE inhibitors. Flushing and arthralgias are common side effects in many medications such as Niaspan or the statins.

39. A: Lasix is a powerful loop diuretic and Mannitol is a powerful osmotic diuretic. They are sometimes used by themselves or together to treat cerebral edema. As diuretics, they help rid the body of fluid, causing serum sodium levels to rise. They have minimal direct effect on serum glucose, white blood cell count, and platelets.

40. C: Avoid areas of low-oxygen concentration
Areas of low-oxygen concentration (as in high altitudes) should be avoided because they may lead to sickle cell crisis. Applying *warm* compresses, not cold, can stimulate circulation and reduce discomfort to the affected area. Fluids should be encouraged to rehydrate cells. Strenuous exercise, emotional stress, cigarette smoking, and alcohol can induce a sickle cell crisis.

41. C: Administering I.V. fluids and replacing electrolytes
Administration of fluids is the top priority for a patient with acute pancreatitis, due to the potential of developing hemodynamic instability and renal failure from decreased renal perfusion. Insertion of an NG and urinary catheter are part of the supportive care of this patient, but not the top priority. Oral intake is discouraged, to decrease pancreatic stimulation for secretion of digestive enzymes.

42. A: The patient is incapacitated and is terminally ill
A Living Will is only appropriate in a situation where the patient is both incapacitated and terminally ill. A grown child with Medical Power of Attorney only makes decisions with the

guidance of the attending physician when the patient is hopelessly terminal and unresponsive.

43. B: Graves' disease is caused by an autoimmune response that causes the body to produce excessive thyroid hormone. Symptoms can include tachycardia, unintentional weight loss, tremor, irregular menstrual cycles, and bulging eyes. Many things can cause hyperthyroidism, but Graves' disease is the most common cause. Treatments include propylthiouracil and methimazole (Tapazole).

44. D: Diabetes does not cause anemia. Diabetics have higher levels of blood sugar since their pancreas produces insufficient or no insulin, which can lead to obesity. High levels of blood glucose stimulate systemic inflammation and atherosclerosis formation causing a multitude of other pathologies. Atherosclerotic plaques decrease the lumen of blood vessels causing hypertension, blindness, and renal insufficiency.

45. C: There are three stages in the nurse-client therapeutic relationship: orientation, exploration, and termination. In the first stage the nurse and client establish limitations, boundaries, trust, and rapport. In the second stage the nurse and client should be able to identify problems or issues and potential solutions to those issues. The nurse may offer assistance or teach the client coping mechanisms in order to face some of the issues. The nurse may assume different roles in order to help the client deal with the stressful situation he/she is facing. In the last phase, the relationship is terminated upon discharge or transfer. The goal of the third stage is the resolution of the client's issues and/or achieving acceptance of the problems and ways to cope with them.

46. C: Tardive dyskinesia is the abnormal involuntary movement of the tongue and/or lower face. It is a common side effect of older anti-psychotic medications such as Haldol. If it occurs, a psychiatrist should be consulted to discuss the possibility of slowly weaning the patient off of Haldol and placing the patient on one of the newer anti-psychotic medications which generally have a lower incidence of causing tardive dyskinesia.

47. C: The current recommendation in the United States is to get screened 10 years prior to the age at which a first-degree relative was diagnosed with colon cancer. If no risk factors are present, then it is recommended to obtain a colonoscopy by 50 years of age. Since she had no significant family history, then her first colonoscopy should be when she is 50 years old, which is 10 years from now.

48. B: Naloxone is an opiate antagonist and will reverse the effects of the medication.

49. B: From the choices given, patients with esophageal varices have the highest risk of bleeding so they are the least desirable patients to be given Plavix. Patients with ischemic strokes, heart attacks, and cardiac or neurosurgical procedures are commonly given Plavix post-operatively. Plavix prevents platelets from sticking together too readily, which helps to prevent against clot formation.

50. D: Jaundice is not caused by an overdose of atropine. Common side effects seen with atropine overdose include fever, blurred vision, diaphoresis, flushing, and altered mental status. A common mnemonic for atropine overdose is "hot as a hare, blind as a bat, dry as a bone, red as a beet, and mad as a hatter." Currently symptomatic relief and fluid hydration are the only treatments for atropine overdose.

51. D: Tetralogy of Fallot is the most common type of cyanotic congenital heart defect. The most common congenital heart defect is ventricular septal defect. Tricuspid atresia is one of the most uncommon cyanotic congenital heart defects. Aortic stenosis may be congenital, but is usually acquired later on in life.

52. C: Sickle cell disease is an autosomal recessive disease that causes red blood cells to be abnormally shaped. This can cause chronic anemia, renal failure, cardiac arrest, splenomegaly, stroke, heart attack, and pulmonary embolus. There is no cure. It does not cause esophageal varices. Esophageal varices are dilated veins in the esophagus commonly caused by cirrhosis due to alcoholism.

53. C: Lexapro is an SSRI (selective serotonin reuptake inhibitor) that is used to treat anxiety and depression. Levoxyl is a synthetic thyroid hormone used in the treatment of hypothyroidism. Haldol is an anti-psychotic medication used to treat bipolar disorder, schizophrenia, and Tourette's syndrome. Keppra is an anticonvulsant primarily used in the treatment and prophylaxis of seizures.

54. B: The patient's son is understandably grief-stricken over his mother's stroke and would benefit from talking to the social worker who could arrange a meeting with a grief counselor. Educating the patient's son about the pathophysiology behind a stroke may help him later on, but is inappropriate and unnecessary while he is in acute distress. Educating the patient's son on the stages of grief should be left to the grief counselor and social worker; it will not help him while he is currently in distress. Calling the police is unnecessary since the patient's son did not harm or threaten to harm himself, the nurse, or others.

55. C: Desmopressin is another name for antidiuretic hormone (ADH) used in treating those who have diabetes insipidus. Diabetes insipidus is caused by insufficient ADH which causes the body to conserve little if any water. Kayexalate is used for patients with hyperkalemia. Insulin is used in patients with hyperglycemia usually caused by diabetes mellitus. Decadron is a steroid used to treat certain types of skin disorders and autoimmune diseases.

56. B: This patient is most likely suffering from Steven-Johnson syndrome caused by a reaction he's having to penicillin. It is a reaction of the skin and mucous membranes to medication or to a medical condition. It begins with nonspecific upper respiratory infection symptoms and then progresses to dermal manifestations. It can be life threatening if not treated immediately and adequately. Cushing syndrome is caused by too much cortisol causing symptoms such as buffalo hump or posterior cervical fat pad, swelling of the face, myalgias, unintentional weight gain, irregular menses, striae, hirsutism, hyperglycemia, and bone loss. Guillain-Barré syndrome is an autoimmune disease causing muscle weakness or paralysis. Turner Syndrome is a genetic condition where females are missing all or part of an X chromosome. Some of the symptoms may include infertility, amenorrhea, short stature, and webbed neck.

57. C: This patient has infective endocarditis caused by her drug use. Endocarditis causes a number of symptoms, but the most classic are fever, chills, and diaphoresis. Common causes are indwelling triple lumen catheters or PICC lines, dental procedures, and IV drug abuse with contaminated needles. The sign indicating the diagnosis is the presence of Janeway

lesions. These lesions are painful erythematous areas on the palms and soles which are only caused by endocarditis.

58. B: Levothyroxine or Synthroid is a synthetic thyroid hormone used to treat Hashimoto's thyroiditis, which causes hypothyroidism. Propylthiouracil and methimazole (Tapazole) are used to treat hyperthyroidism caused by Graves' disease. Lantus is a type of exogenous insulin used to treat those with diabetes.

59. C: Clindamycin, gentamicin, and penicillin are not medications that would be used in the treatment of tuberculosis. There are a multitude of medications used to treat tuberculosis; they are used in a variety of combination therapies. The more common medications are isoniazid, rifampin, pyrazinamide, and ethambutol. Less common drug remedies include amikacin, ethionamide, moxifloxacin, para-aminosalicylic acid, and streptomycin. Affected patients are usually on multiple medications for six months or longer.

60. B: Thrush is a yeast infection seen in patients who are poorly controlled diabetics, those who have been on long-term steroids or antibiotics, and immunocompromised patients. It is similar in appearance to euplasia, except in cases of thrush the white lesions may be scraped off. The causes of leukoplakia are unknown, but it is commonly seen in alcoholics and those who smoke or chew tobacco. Parotitis is an infection of the parotid gland which can produce facial swelling and pain. Gingivostomatitis is an infection of the mouth and gums appearing as painful sores.

61. B: Proventil, Xopenex, and Ventolin are short-acting beta-2 bronchodilators. These medications are some of the first-line agents in treating an acute asthma exacerbation. Mucinex will help with excessive congestion seen with upper respiratory infections, but should not be used in an acute asthma exacerbation. Singulair is a leukotriene inhibitor used to prevent asthma attacks, but will not work quickly enough to alleviate symptoms in an acute asthma attack. Therefore during an acute asthma exacerbation, other medications should be used. Augmentin is an antibiotic that will not be effective when treating asthma unless an underlying infection is present.

62. D: Paraphimosis is when the foreskin of the penis cannot be reduced back to its original position. If it cannot be done at bedside with conservative methods then surgical intervention may be necessary. Gangrene may occur if left untreated. The other choices given are not side effects or complications resulting from paraphimosis. Mastitis is the inflammation of the breasts, which is common in lactating mothers.

63. D: G6PD deficiency is an X-linked recessive hereditary disease where the defect of this enzyme causes red blood cells to break down prematurely. It is much more prevalent in males than females. It is the most common enzyme defect in humans. Many types of foods (such as legumes and artificial food coloring), medications (NSAIDs, aspirin, and sulfa drugs), and environmental triggers (moth balls, pollen, and henna), can cause acute exacerbations. The only treatment for this disease is to avoid known triggers as much as possible.

64. B: Sickle cell disease is an autosomal recessive genetic blood disorder caused by a defect on chromosome 11. Patients who have only one recessive allele have sickle cell trait; they are usually asymptomatic and do not suffer the same medical complications as those with the disease. Sickle cell disease increases the risk of stroke, heart attack, pulmonary

hypertension, skin ulcers, priapism, as well as other health problems. Sickle cell disease does not increase the risk for diabetes.

65. B: The Joint Commission defines a sentinel event as an unexpected injury or complication, not due to the patient's primary diagnosis, which may or may not cause the death of the patient. The patient aspirating because the hospital staff mistakenly gave her the wrong diet was the first sentinel event. The patient dying from anaphylaxis because the hospital gave her an antibiotic to which she had a documented allergy was the second sentinel event.

66. A: The patient had one sentinel event during the hospital stay. The Joint Commission defines a sentinel event as an unexpected injury or complication which may or may not cause the death of the patient and is not due to the patient's primary diagnosis. The patient received Nimotop by the incorrect route which caused severe hypotension causing the stroke.

67. C: Fruity-smelling breath is a sign of ketoacidosis, which would occur in hyperglycemic patients. Signs and symptoms of hypoglycemia include altered mental status, nausea, vomiting, diaphoresis, palpitations, polyphagia, tremor, weakness, and in rare cases, seizures. Receiving sugar either by mouth or IV in the event the patient is lethargic will correct hypoglycemia.

68. C: Chvostek's sign is positive when tapping on a patient's zygoma induces facial twitching. It is commonly seen in those with hypocalcemia. A common mnemonic to remember the signs and symptoms of hypercalcemia includes "stones, bones, groans, and psychiatric overtones." Hypercalcemia can cause stones to form in the renal and biliary tracts, bony pain, abdominal pain caused by constipation, and psychiatric symptoms such as anxiety, depression, and cognitive dysfunction.

69. D. This pattern of pain—severe epigastric pain radiating to the back—that is exacerbated by lying flat or walking is consistent with pancreatitis. Generally, the upper abdomen is tender but without rigidity or guarding, which may be present with other disorders. Abdominal distention and jaundice may occur in some patients. Fever to 39° C is common as is tachycardia and pallor. Serum amylase and serum lipase may be elevated up to 3 times normal values within 24 hours, and leukocytosis (10,000 to 30,000) may be evident.

70. D: MRIs are generally contraindicated in those with pacemakers or implantable metal devices. MRI (magnetic resonance imaging) scans work by using magnets. These magnets can cause pacemaker dysfunction and may actually pull the pacemaker out of a patient's chest causing hemorrhage, cardiac arrest, and potentially death. Currently, some pacemakers are being created that are MRI compatible. However, unless the patient carries a card that verifies that their pacemaker is MRI compatible, MRIs should be avoided in that patient.

71. C: Shaving the patient's chest is the next appropriate step since the electrodes will not adhere on their own. The nurse should explain to the patient that patches of the chest need to be shaved in order for the electrodes to adhere to the patient. Placing the electrodes on the back instead of on the chest will result in an inaccurate and likely unusable EKG. A 2D echo will take longer to obtain than an EKG and should not be used in a patient who may be

having an acute myocardial infarction. Forgoing the EKG just because the electrodes will not stick is inappropriate.

72. B: Acting out the surgical procedure is the most inappropriate because the gestures the nurse is using may confuse the patient. In order for the patient to understand what she is signing, the nurse needs to be as clear as possible. This includes facing the patient when speaking, speaking in a loud clear voice, and allowing the patient to read the consents themselves. This way the patient understands what procedure she will be undergoing and the possible complications that may occur.

73. D: The administration of D50 is used for patients who have hypoglycemia. D50 will only worsen hyperglycemia, causing further complications. Lantus is a long-acting anti-hyperglycemic medication; in acute hyperglycemia short-acting insulin should be used as well. IV fluid hydration is important because patients in ketoacidosis are usually dehydrated. The IV fluids help correct the dehydration and improve electrolyte abnormalities that may have occurred because of the dehydration. Kayexalate binds to the potassium in the blood and it is excreted out of the body via bowel movements. This is important because hyperglycemia causes ketoacidosis; the acidosis is improved/resolved by ridding the body of some of the potassium.

74. B: CT angiogram would be contraindicated. In cases of allergy to IV dye, patients may be prepped beforehand. The prep includes steroids and Benadryl. In cases of severe allergies such as anaphylaxis, the risks and benefits of getting the test must be weighed by the attending physician. Anaphylaxis is defined as a serious allergic reaction that causes the rapid appearance of signs and symptoms which may ultimately result in death. Sometimes an MRI with gadolinium may be ordered instead, since gadolinium has a different composition than the contrast used in CT scans.

75. B: Females have a lower risk for cardiovascular artery disease (CAD) than their male counterparts. Other risk factors include high cholesterol, stress level, weight, and activity. Even if the high blood pressure and diabetes are controlled, the patient is still at an increased risk for CAD. However, those with controlled diabetes and hypertension are at less of a risk than patients who have uncontrolled comorbidities.

76. A: Stabilizing the patient's airway is the most crucial first step in stabilizing the patient. Her oxygenation is only 76% on NRB – the patient is not receiving sufficient oxygen and will go into cardiac arrest and develop neurological compromise if this is not reversed. Anaphylaxis is defined as a serious allergic reaction that causes the rapid appearance of signs and symptoms which may ultimately result in death. The patient does need to be given Zofran for the vomiting and Benadryl for the rash, but these can be given after the patient is safely intubated. CPR is not warranted in this case because the patient still has a patent airway, the patient is not unconscious, and no cardiac arrhythmia is mentioned.

77. B: Urinary and bowel retention does not occur with anaphylaxis. Anaphylaxis is defined as a serious allergic reaction that causes the rapid appearance of signs and symptoms which may ultimately result in death. Bowel or bladder incontinence is usually associated with anaphylaxis. Respiratory distress leading to failure and cardiac arrest are two of the most serious complications that may occur. Angioedema is the appearance of facial swelling which is usually not life-threatening and may be treated with steroids.

78. A: Oxytocin has many roles, but in childbirth it helps to initiate and strengthen uterine contractions that will help expel the fetus and the afterbirth. After labor it is given to the mother again to help the uterus contract back to its prior size, which helps decrease the risk of postpartum hemorrhage. It has little to do with preventing jaundice and does not decrease pain. If anything it increases pain since it increases contractions. RhoGAM is used to prevent hemolytic disease of the newborn, not oxytocin.

79. C: A nurse should be wearing gloves at all times no matter what diagnosis the patient may have. Since the patient is on contact precautions due to *C. difficile* colitis, a gown needs to be worn whenever the nurse enters the patient's room. Prior to leaving the room, the nurse should remove the gown. The same gown should never be worn in another patient's room because the nurse may infect the healthy patient. Since the patient likely has profuse watery diarrhea, a face mask with a shield should be worn to help prevent accidental body fluid exposure. A cap may be worn, but is not necessary.

80. C: Von Willebrand disease is a hereditary bleeding disorder caused by factor VIII clotting deficiency. It is a much milder form of hemophilia. Parkinson's disease destroys dopamine-producing neurons in the substantia nigra, and causes motor symptoms (dyskinesia, tremor, rigidity) as well as cognitive symptoms. Turner syndrome is a genetic condition where females are missing all or part of an X chromosome. Some of the symptoms may include infertility, amenorrhea, short stature, and webbed neck. Down syndrome is a genetic condition where there is a chromosomal abnormality on chromosome 21. Some signs of Down syndrome may include broad forehead and tongue, slanted eyes, small ears, and cognitive and cardiac defects.

81. A. One of the barriers to adequate pain management is nurses' preconceptions about physiological and emotional responses to pain and what a patient in pain should look like. Some patients moan and cry while others show little outward sign of pain, but pain is what the patient says it is, and if a patient requests pain medication for severe pain, then the nurse should give the opioid. A patient may try to not to show pain to family members or friends even when the patient is very uncomfortable.

82. C: Deep vein thrombus is the most likely diagnosis. It will usually present with calf pain and/or swelling. In approximately 30 percent of cases, the patient will also have a positive Homan's sign. Pain is elicited with passive sudden dorsiflexion of the foot. Phlebitis is the inflammation and occasionally thrombosis of a superficial vein. Patients usually present with unilateral lower extremity erythema with or without swelling and a palpable cord, which is the affected vein. This is usually preceded by trauma. The Homan's sign is negative. Compartment syndrome is a life-threatening condition which compromises the blood flow to the affected extremity. This could result in amputation if not treated emergently. The extremity is initially erythematous, but then turns cyanotic as blood flow diminishes. The pulses of the affected extremity are diminished or absent. This condition is usually preceded by trauma. The Homan's sign is negative. Raynaud's disease is caused by the body's abnormal response to cold weather and to stress. The body significantly decreases the blood flow to the extremities, causing pallor or cyanosis and paresthesias. This occurs in bilateral extremities. The Homan's sign is negative.

83. A: Alcohol can cause many complications in a fetus, but it is not a risk factor in developing listeriosis. Listeriosis is spread through contaminated food, milk, soil, and water. Therefore, avoiding unpasteurized milk is recommended. It is also recommended to

thoroughly wash produce, cook meat and fish prior to eating it, and to limit processed foods such as hot dogs and deli meats during pregnancy. Hot dogs and deli meats may be contaminated after they are cooked and prior to being packaged. Pregnant women infected with Listeria may only exhibit mild symptoms, but the disease may result in death of the fetus.

84. C. It's very important that an impermeable covering be placed over the insertion site until the chest tube can be reinserted to prevent air from sucking into the pleural cavity. If no plastic or petroleum gauze dressing is available, the nurse can cover the insertion site with a clean gloved hand while calling for assistance. The physician must be notified as soon as the insertion site is secured. The patient's arterial blood gases should be assessed as soon as possible.

85. A. A potassium level of 3.2 mEq/L indicates hypokalemia, which increases the risk of digoxin toxicity. Immediate treatment includes withholding digoxin (the number of doses or the need for reduction in dosage depends on the severity of the reaction as well as the cause). With hypokalemia, potassium supplement should be administered as well as supportive therapy, such as acetaminophen for headache and an antidiarrheal. The digoxin antidote, digoxin immune Fab, is not routinely given but may be administered if indicated, usually because of severe toxicity with hyperkalemia, severe cardiac dysrhythmias, or digoxin overdose.

86. A: Parkinson's disease destroys dopamine-producing neurons in the substantia nigra, and causes motor symptoms (dyskinesia, tremor, rigidity) as well as cognitive symptoms. Approximately 80 percent of the substantia nigra is destroyed prior to the onset of symptoms. There is no cure, but medications can be prescribed to help alleviate the severity of the symptoms.

87. D: Addison's disease is caused by a lack of cortisol. Giving cortisol exogenously helps alleviate the disease's symptoms. Common presenting symptoms include hypotension and hyperpigmentation. It is caused by lack of an adrenal gland, an adrenal gland that produces insufficient amounts of cortisol, or a previously normal adrenal gland that has become damaged due to disease or trauma.

88. B: Though it is preferred that the power of attorney sign consents in person, consent may be given over the phone, but it must be witnessed by at least two nurses. This is done to ensure that the patient's identity is correct, the procedure and associated risks are understood, and the opportunity for questions is provided.

89. D: The patient most likely has benign prostatic hypertrophy (BPH) which becomes more common in men as they age. A coude catheter is a slim curved catheter specifically designed for those with BPH. A Foley catheter is more rigid and is thicker. A nasogastric tube and a Dobhoff (a thinner, more flexible nasogastric tube) play no role in the treatment of urinary retention.

90. C: Since the NGT is halfway out, the NGT should be pulled out and a new one should be inserted. A chest x-ray should be obtained to ensure that the NGT is in the correct position prior to restarting tube feeds and medications. Though this may delay the administration of medications, it is the safest for the patient. The NGT is often accidentally placed in the left mainstem bronchus or in the esophagus; if tube feeds and/or medications are given without

checking the placement, the patient could aspirate and potentially die. If a patient is ordered to receive medications and tube feeds through the NGT, a nurse should never take it upon him/herself to attempt to start oral feedings.

91. C: Patients should limit their calcium/dairy intake since most stones are composed of calcium oxalate. To prevent calcium deficiency, patients are recommended to take calcium supplements. Remaining adequately hydrated is the most important recommendation to patients who have had several episodes of nephrolithiasis. Reducing protein intake can also help prevent kidney stones. Animal protein contains purines which break down into uric acid. Kidney stones are not always composed of calcium oxalate; sometimes they are composed of uric acid. Decreasing one's sodium intake can help prevent dehydration, which may precipitate reoccurrence of stone formation.

92. B: Surgical debridement is generally not a treatment modality for stage II decubitus ulcers unless secondary infection is present. Stage I decubitus ulcers present as non-blanching erythema without skin break. Stage II decubitus ulcers invade the epidermis and sometimes the dermis of the skin. Stage III decubitus ulcers invade the subcutaneous fascia. Stage IV decubitus ulcers invade the muscles and tendons and sometimes erode the bone. Stages III and IV often require multiple treatment modalities, including surgery. Stages I and II are usually treated more conservatively and will resolve if taken care of quickly and appropriately.

93. D: Ménière's disease is caused by a dysfunction in the inner ear causing episodes of vertigo. Motion sickness medications and antiemetic medications such as Antivert and Zofran, respectively, may provide symptomatic relief of vertigo symptoms. Diuretics such as Lasix may be given to normalize the fluid in the inner ear. Haloperidol is an anti-psychotic medication that is not used in the treatment of Ménière's disease.

94. A: A colonoscopy is a screening test to detect pathology that may already exist in an asymptomatic patient. Performing a beta HCG on a patient to monitor the reoccurrence of choriocarcinoma is another example of secondary prevention. Primary prevention helps to prevent the pathology before it exists. Obtaining a vaccination to help protect against cervical cancer is an example of primary prevention. Tertiary prevention is aimed at helping alleviate pain and preventing secondary complications from a pathology/infection/disease that has already occurred. Obtaining radiation and chemotherapy in a patient with lung cancer is an example.

95. C: The open incision should be addressed first. The wound should be covered to help control the bleeding and the surgeon should be called immediately. An open incision increases the risk for infection and the bleeding needs to be controlled. Covering the wound will help, but any time there is a wound dehiscence the attending should be notified. The pain and nausea should be treated next, followed by the decubitus ulcer.

96. B: The Joint Commission recommends at least two forms of identification (e.g., a medical record number and a name or a name and a birth date) prior to performing a procedure or administering medications. This helps prevent mistakes and protects the patients. In cases of surgical intervention, the operative site should also be clearly marked as well as using two forms of identification.

97. D: The appendectomy patient should be seen last since this patient is sleeping and does not currently have a complaint. Though recent post-operative patients should usually be seen first, this patient is the most stable patient from the choices provided. The patient with the subdural hematoma with a neurological change should be evaluated first. The psychiatric patient complaining of chest pain should be evaluated second. Even though this patient has a history of psychiatric issues and his vitals are stable, there could be a serious underlying pathology causing this patient's chest pain. The femur fracture patient, although uncomfortable, will not have a change in his prognosis if pain medication is delayed a few minutes while the nurse examines another patient. This patient should be evaluated third.

98. A: Sending repeat serum potassium is the most appropriate intervention. Since the specimen was hemolyzed it is expected to be high. However, it is important that the nurse find out the patient's actual potassium level. A patient may have elevated serum potassium at baseline, but since the specimen was hemolyzed there is no way to know how high the level is. No interventions should be performed until the repeat potassium is resulted.

99. C: An employee should never ignore an incident involving chemical or body fluid exposure. It is dangerous for the nurse and for the patients he is caring for. The nurse should stop working immediately and have someone call the nurse manager while he irrigates the eye. Afterwards the nurse should go to Employee Health to report the incident and determine if the injury requires further attention.

100. A: The chest tube should be placed on suction until the air leak resolves. If the air leak is coming from inside of the chest it means that the lung/airway is not sealed. It is more difficult for the lung to reinflate if there is an air leak. The tubing should never be clamped indefinitely. Intrathoracic air may reaccumulate and result in a pneumothorax. Not intervening is not appropriate. If there is something wrong with an indwelling drain it needs to be addressed by the patient's nurse. If she/he is unsure of the treatment then the attending physician, resident, or physician assistant should be notified so they can address the problem. A chest tube should never be pulled out unless the attending physician is present and authorizes the nurse to do so.

101. B: In accordance with The Health Insurance Portability and Accountability Act (HIPAA) healthcare providers may not give out patient information to anyone unless the patient gives permission to do so. In the event that the patient is unconscious or otherwise lacking the capacity to give permission, the healthcare provider may give information to the power of attorney or closest known family member (i.e., spouse, parent, child) as long as the family member provides documentation/proof of the relationship status. A person who simply claims to be a family member should not be given information over the phone since there is no way to verify identity. Healthcare providers are not allowed to give information over the phone or in person to anyone other than the power of attorney unless the power of attorney grants permission. Even if the healthcare provider cannot give out information he/she should respond in a respectful manner, unlike how the nurse responded in choice A.

102. B: The supine position is best for a patient who is suffering from a headache post lumbar puncture. This is because the cerebrospinal fluid bathes the brain in fluid, which may alleviate or at least improve the headache. Any other position will exacerbate the headache and increase the risk for developing a subdural hematoma and/or seizure. The mainstays of treatment for a spinal headache include oral analgesics, rest, and IV fluids.

Epidural blood patches are used to treat CSF leaks that may cause persistent headaches refractory to conservative measures.

103. D: This is the most appropriate answer because the nurse is acknowledging the patient's struggle to remember and is helping him formulate a plan to be more compliant. Choices A and B are inappropriate and unprofessional responses. While the patient should be educated on the risks of noncompliance, it should be done in a caring, compassionate, and professional manner. While choice C is not completely inappropriate, the nurse should be encouraging him to be compliant with all medications and not just some of them.

104. A. Because potassium-sparing diuretics markedly increase the risk of hyperkalemia in patients with chronic kidney disease, they are usually used only with patients who have persistent hypokalemia or hypertension. Risk is highest in patients whose glomerular filtration rate is less than 30 mL/min/1.73 m² and are also receiving ACEI or ARBs. Dosages should begin low and be increased slowly. Electrolyte levels must be monitored frequently. Hyporeninemic hypoaldosteronism is a contraindication for the use of potassium-sparing diuretics.

105. C: Performing a diverting colostomy in a patient with a stage III decubitus ulcer would be a tertiary prevention because its aim is to prevent secondary complications (i.e., infection of an ulcer) from a pathology/infection/disease that has already occurred. Stage III decubitus ulcers invade the subcutaneous fascia. They are treated with a multitude of treatments including surgery. Surgery would be indicated in this case because the ulcer is close to the rectum and if the ulcer is exposed to stool/urine it has a high chance of becoming infected. Secondary intervention's goal is to detect pathology that may already exist in an asymptomatic patient. Performing a mammogram is an example of secondary prevention. Primary prevention helps to prevent the pathology before it exists. Obtaining a vaccination to help protect against cervical cancer is an example of primary prevention.

106. A: A banana bag is typically composed of a multivitamin, thiamine, folic acid, and electrolytes. The name derives from its bright yellow appearance. It is given to patients with acute alcohol intoxication to correct electrolyte imbalances and nutrient deficiencies. Alcoholic patients are chronically malnourished and have deficiencies in both thiamine and folic acid. It is also used to help rehydrate the patient. Although banana bags may help decrease the severity of a hangover, they may not necessarily prevent a hangover.

107. C: Synthroid is a synthetic thyroid hormone taken exogenously to help treat hypothyroidism. The patient's thyroid is not making sufficient thyroid hormone, which can be due to a multitude of reasons, and if this is not corrected severe complications can occur. Signs and symptoms of hypothyroidism may include bradycardia, dry skin, hair loss, unintentional weight gain due to slowed metabolism, short stature, and neurological abnormalities.

108. A. The two most commonly used drugs to treat delirium are lorazepam and haloperidol. Anticholinergics, such as benztropine, may trigger delirium, especially in older adults. Delirium has similar symptoms as dementia; but with delirium the symptoms tend to fluctuate, so patients may have both periods of lucidity and profound confusion. Delirium may be triggered by many conditions, such as trauma, depression, surgery, untreated pain, and electrolyte imbalance. A patient's attention deficit may be noted if the patient is unable to count backward from 1 to 20 or spell his first name backward.

109. D: Limiting/avoiding caffeine would help with stress incontinence. Caffeine acts as a diuretic, which would make patients have to go to the bathroom more often and will only exacerbate their condition. Taking frequent bathroom breaks helps prevent unwanted leakage. Kegel exercises serve to strengthen the pelvic floor muscles and help prevent urine incontinence. Avoiding alcohol, which also acts as a diuretic, may be helpful to this patient.

110. A: A patient should never be told that he has to go home, or to a rehab, or to a long-term care facility. The medical team may make suggestions to the patient and family, but the patient should never be forced to go to another facility. Since the patient does have difficulties with carrying out activities of daily life, a home health aide would be helpful. His wife/primary caregiver should be educated on how to assist the patient to take care of himself. If the burden of assistance is too great on the family/primary caregiver, rehab is advisable before sending the patient home.

111. D: While in the acute grieving process after just learning that a loved one is going to die, it is inappropriate to ask about organ donation. In most cases it is also not nurse that should approach the family, but an organ procurement organization. The family needs time to let the news sink in before the sensitive topic about organ donation should be broached. Since the family is agitated and yelling obscenities, it would not be considered inappropriate if the nurse asked them respectfully to lower their voices or go to a private family room to grieve. Closing the door temporarily to give the patient's family some additional privacy to grieve is appropriate. Asking the family if they would like a religious leader to be called is appropriate, as many religions have end-of-life rites that are performed. The patient's family should always be asked whether or not they want a religious leader to be called since some people do not adhere to religious beliefs.

112. A: If the airway is patent, but has ineffective clearance, and LMA would not help, as it would make an even smaller airway to have to keep clear. A patient should be placed in a sitting position or in reverse Trendelenburg so that their airway remains patent. A patient with ineffective airway clearance placed in the supine position is at greater risk for aspiration. Chest percussion, medications such as Mucinex or Robinul that help decrease secretions, use of the incentive spirometer, and nebulizer treatments are all methods in which nurses can assist patients to clear their airways.

113. B: The patient may be abused and/or neglected by the family, and a social worker should be involved for further investigation. It is suspicious that an elderly woman is living with her family and no one has seen her or checked in on her in almost a week. Though an assisted living facility will most likely be needed, developing a discharge plan is premature at this time. Sending pictures of the patient to the police is inappropriate and unethical. In accordance with The Health Insurance Portability and Accountability Act (HIPAA) healthcare providers may not give out patient information to anyone unless the patient or designated power of attorney gives permission to do so. If the social worker needs the police to get involved, he/she will arrange it. It is imperative, however, that the nurse document all of the injuries and physical findings in detail. The nurse should only ask questions pertinent to the case; the patient's family members should never be interrogated by the medical staff regarding suspected abuse or neglect. The police may question the family with lawyers and a social worker present.

114. A: Primary prevention helps to prevent the pathology before it exists. Tetanus immunizations help prevent against *Clostridium tetani* infections. Secondary intervention's goal is to detect pathology that may already exist in an asymptomatic patient. Performing a colonoscopy on a regular basis will not prevent cancer; its goal is early detection. Tertiary prevention's aim is to prevent secondary complications from a pathology/infection/disease that has already occurred.

115. C: The patient should receive her next tetanus shot in five years since tetanus immunizations are good for ten years. If the patient was unsure of her vaccination status, a tetanus shot would be given during this hospital visit as a precautionary measure. Tetanus immunizations help prevent against *Clostridium tetani* infections such as lockjaw.

116. A: Malaria is transmitted by infected mosquitoes in tropical and subtropical areas. It causes a variety of symptoms which include nausea, vomiting, fever, myalgias, splenomegaly, hematuria, neurological compromise, seizures, coma, and death. It is diagnosed by peripheral blood smear. Antimalarial medications such as mefloquine, atovaquone, and chloroquine as well as antibiotics such as doxycycline are used to treat the disease.

117. A. When the Passy-Muir valve is placed on a tracheostomy tube, the cuff must be completely deflated. If mechanical ventilation is used, the tidal volume should also be increased. The Passy-Muir valve is a one-way valve that opens on inhalation so that air can enter the lungs and closes on exhalation, forcing the air over the vocal chords and out the mouth instead of out the tracheostomy tube. The valve may be used to help the patient regain normal breathing patterns, improve swallowing, and decrease the risk of aspiration.

118. D: Penicillin is the treatment of choice for patients who have had syphilis for less than one year. Syphilis is a sexually transmitted disease similar to gonorrhea and chlamydia that if caught early is easily treated and has no sequelae. If left untreated syphilis can lead to meningitis, stroke, neurological compromise, deafness, stillbirth, and death.

119. B. The primary concern with combining these drugs is that hydrochlorothiazide can interfere with the action of antidiabetic agents, decreasing hypoglycemic effects; so patients may develop hyperglycemia and should be advised to careful monitor their blood glucose levels when beginning treatment since the dosage for the antidiabetic agent may need to be increased. Patients should also be advised to avoid licorice, which may cause increased potassium loss, and alcohol, which may cause orthostatic hypotension.

120. B. Celiac disease results in malabsorption of folate and iron, so patients are often anemic. Additionally, damage to the lining of the small intestines from gluten sensitivity interferes with absorption of fats and calcium, so patients may exhibit osteomalacia and bone pain and steatorrhea. Celiac disease is an autoimmune disorder in which antibodies to gluten in the diet cause inflammation and damage to intestinal villi. Patients must be maintained on a strict gluten-free diet. Gluten is found in some grains, such as wheat.

121. B: A patient who has a terminal disease or injury with severely depressed mental status may be made CMO by the family/power of attorney, which allows the healthcare team to assist in the process of dying, but ensures that the patient is made comfortable. This entails withholding life-saving measures/medications, supplemental oxygen, CPR, IV fluids, and tube feeds/food.

122. A: The patient's needs supersede the day nurse's anger. While the night nurse may not have been diligent in her care of this patient, it is now the day nurse's duty to attend to this patient's needs. It would be appropriate to call the nurse manager later and voice his concern about the night nurse's care, but the patient should be taken care of first. Since there is no current conflict with the night nurse, a conflict resolution meeting is unnecessary at this time. It is inappropriate and unprofessional for the day nurse to call, e-mail, or text the night nurse to reprimand her. If he feels that strongly about the incident, a conflict resolution meeting can be scheduled with a supervisor as the mediator.

123. D: Think of the mnemonic ABC (Airway, Breathing, Circulation) as a way to prioritize things that need to be addressed. All three of these issues need to be addressed quickly to maximize the patient's chance for a good outcome. If the patient is mildly hypoxic then the first thing the nurse needs to do is give the patient supplemental oxygen. The nurse should not prepare for chest tube placement unless a chest x-ray shows a pneumothorax. If the patient was a trauma patient with penetrating chest trauma and/or there was high suspicion for a pneumothorax, then preparations can be made for placement after the patient is stabilized. A history and physical as well as an EKG should be performed after the patient is stabilized.

124. B. Fluid intelligence is the ability to see relationships, reason, and think abstractly—all qualities needed to facilitate learning. Older adults tend to have altered time perception so that time seems to pass more quickly than when they were younger, so they may focus more on the here and now rather than on future needs. Other changes include increased test anxiety, decreased short-term (rather than long-term) memory, increased processing and reaction time, and persistence of stimuli (confusing older learning with newer).

125. C: One or both nurses should report the change in neurological exam to the attending, resident, or licensed independent practitioner (LIP). The night nurse should not be reported since the change in neurological status happened at change of shift. If the neurological change occurred earlier in the night shift and the night nurse did not report it to the attending, resident, or LIP, then the night nurse should be reported. The day nurse should not wait another hour to evaluate the neurological change. As soon as a change occurs, it should be reported so that the attending physician can determine whether or not further intervention is required. It is illegal and unethical for a nurse to change the documented physical exam overnight to match the patient's current exam.

126. A: Tissue plasminogen activator (tPA) is a very strong clot-busting medication given to patients with stroke or acute myocardial infarctions. After being given this medication patients generally should not receive blood thinners, anti-platelet medications, or lines since their risk of bleeding is very high. This period lasts for approximately 24 hours until the medication is out of the patient's system. Since the patient just received tPA, a Foley catheter would be contraindicated. The patient is cognizant so the nurse should offer a bed pan often to help prevent the patient from soiling herself. A nephrology consult is inappropriate for urinary incontinence. A urology consult may be needed, not nephrology. Also, the urology consult may not be needed immediately. The patient's incontinence caused by the stroke may improve. Having a recent tPA patient with moderate motor deficits ambulate to the commode, even with assistance, is dangerous and inappropriate.

127. C: Keppra is used to prevent and treat seizures. Medications such as heparin, Lovenox, Arixtra, or Coumadin may help prevent deep vein thromboses. Medications such as calcium channel blockers, beta blockers, and ACE inhibitors may help improve high blood pressure. Medications like senna, Colace, or Dulcolax may help regulate bowel movements.

128. D: The nurse should call the attending, resident, or licensed independent practitioner (LIP) and get hold parameters on this medication. The patient's blood pressure is low, and giving the patient Norvasc can cause the blood pressure to become dangerously low. Though it is appropriate to hold the Norvasc, the nurse should speak to the attending/resident/LIP and get an order to hold it. Giving double the dose of Norvasc without an order is dangerous, inappropriate, and unethical. Since the Norvasc doesn't have hold parameters, it would not be the nurse's fault necessarily if the Norvasc was given, but the nurse should always use his/her judgment and assess a patient's physical exam and vital signs prior to administering medications.

129. A. The femoral nerve may become damaged during the fem-pop bypass procedure, resulting in numbness and tingling in the anterior and medial aspects of the thigh. The femoral nerve activates muscles used to extend the leg and move the hips, so damage may impair mobility (depending upon the degree). The damage may occur as direct injury or from compression related to edema and inflammation. The symptoms may recede over time, although some patients will need physical therapy to strengthen muscles.

130. C: The patient who is about to go to the OR should be seen first to make sure that all of the necessary paperwork is in order, all pertinent medications were given or withheld, the patient is being kept NPO, the patient doesn't have any unanswered questions, his vitals are normal/stable, and there are no abnormalities with his labs. The rest of the patients are stable.

131. B: A mnemonic for remembering the common causes of post-operative fever is the five Ws: **w**ind (atelectasis, aspiration, pneumonia), **w**ater (urinary tract infection), **w**alking (deep vein thrombus), **w**ound (wound infection), **w**hat the physician caused (drug fever, line infection). Wind is most likely to cause a fever POD 1–2, water is most likely to cause a fever POD 3–5, walking is the most likely to cause a fever POD 5–7, wound is the most likely cause of fever POD 5–9, and complications caused by the physician most likely cause a fever after the first week of surgery. In this case choice B is the most appropriate answer.

132. C: The nurse can discuss with the physician the possible need for an endocrinologist but should not discuss tell a patient what they need for care or what to ask a doctor. The patient has incredibly high blood sugar levels (normal level is 70–120) and her anti-hyperglycemic medication regimen should be modified. The nurse should also make sure that the patient's diet is not contributing to the hyperglycemia, and should educate the patient about the risks of persistent hyperglycemia (i.e., renal failure, blindness, neuropathy, stroke, heart attack, and death).

133. D: The patient's blood pressure is dangerously high, and since she already has had a hemorrhagic stroke her blood pressure should be tightly controlled. Although cleaning the patient is important, there are more pressing issues that need to be addressed first. Once the patient is stabilized then she may be cleaned. The patient's nausea may be related to her high blood pressure. High blood pressure can cause nausea and moderate to severe nausea can increase blood pressure. The nausea should be addressed second since dangerously

high blood pressure is more life-threatening than nausea. The patient's blood sugar is normal (normal level 70–120).

134. D. The two types of drugs most commonly implicated in acute hypoglycemia are insulins and sulfonylureas, including glipizide (Glucotrol), which stimulates beta cells in the pancreas to produce more insulin. The hypoglycemic effect of sulfonylureas may be potentiated by other medications that compete for binding sites on albumin. Patients with sulfonylurea-induced hypoglycemia and altered mental status require hospitalization, IV glucose, and careful monitoring, since oral ingestion of carbohydrates alone may not prevent relapses, which may occur for days.

135. A: The nurse should first flush the Foley to make sure the Foley itself is working. If that does not resolve the issue then the attending should be informed. A Foley should never be discontinued without an order. A nephrology consult may be warranted if the patient is in acute renal failure, but the situation should be assessed with the attending prior to ordering a nephrology consult.

136. D: A Texas catheter or a condom catheter fits over the penis of a patient and is not a true line since it is not an indwelling catheter. The other choices given are invasive indwelling catheters that are contraindicated in a recent tPA patient. Tissue plasminogen activator (tPA) is a very strong clot-busting medication given to patients with stroke or acute myocardial infarctions. After being given this medication patients generally should not receive blood thinners, anti-platelet medications, or lines since their risk of bleeding is very high. This period lasts for approximately 24 hours until the medication is out of the patient's system.

137. A: A mnemonic for remembering the common causes of post-operative fever is the five Ws: **w**ind (atelectasis, aspiration, pneumonia), **w**ater (urinary tract infection), **w**alking (deep vein thrombus), **w**ound (wound infection), **w**hat the physician caused (drug fever, line infection). Wind is most likely to cause a fever POD 1–2, water is most likely to cause a fever POD 3–5, walking is the most likely to cause a fever POD 5–7, wound is the most likely cause POD 5–9, and complications caused by the physician most likely cause a fever after the first week of surgery. In this case, choice A is the most appropriate answer.

138. C. These signs and symptoms are characteristic of complete small bowel obstruction (especially not passing flatus for more than 12 hours), the dilated loops of small bowel, and the lack of air in the colon and rectum; so the initial intervention is likely to be exploratory surgery since the risk for ischemia is high. If the blockage is in the proximal part of the small bowel, abdominal distention may not be evident. Laboratory studies, such as the complete blood count and electrolytes, may be normal or abnormal, depending on many factors.

139. B: Keeping patients NPO when they are going through withdrawal isn't usually necessary unless they also have a compromised neurological status that impairs their swallowing. If a patient is being fed, a bland diet is recommended. Benzodiazepines such as Ativan are the treatment of choice because they sedate the patient and alleviate most symptoms. A banana bag is a type of IV fluid which includes folate, thiamine, and a multivitamin, since patients who experience delirium tremens are usually alcoholics and they are generally malnourished. The banana bag's name is derived from its bright yellow color. Many patients going through withdrawal complain of nausea so administering Reglan or Zofran is recommended.

140. A. The patient is exhibiting signs of mild lithium toxicity. Symptoms of mild toxicity are evident with levels 1.5 to 2.5 mEq/L. The therapeutic level of lithium for maintenance therapy is 0.6 to 1.2 mEq/L and 1.0 to 1.5 mEq/L for acute episodes of mania. Lithium has a narrow therapeutic index and levels should be monitored weekly initially and then monthly with patients educated about signs of toxicity. More severe life-threatening symptoms (ECG abnormalities, seizures, coma) can occur with blood levels above 2.5 mEq/L.

141. B: Although pneumonia can be life threatening, this patient is the most stable from the choices given. A patient undergoing a neurological change should be attended to first since this can be due to a number of life-threatening causes: hypoglycemia, intracranial pathology, and hypoxia to name a few. A patient suffering from delirium tremens can suffer seizure, heart attack, stroke, and death. Any time a patient is going to the OR his chart should be checked by the medical team to make sure that all of the necessary paperwork is in order, all pertinent medications were given or withheld, the patient is being kept NPO, the patient doesn't have any unanswered questions, his vitals are normal/stable, and there are no abnormalities with his labs.

142. B: A mnemonic for remembering the common causes of post-operative fever is the five Ws: wind (atelectasis, aspiration, pneumonia), water (urinary tract infection), walking (deep vein thrombus), wound (wound infection), what the physician caused (drug fever, line infection). Wind is most likely to cause a fever POD 1–2, water is most likely to cause a fever POD 3–5, walking is the most likely to cause a fever POD 5–7, wound is the most likely cause POD 5–9, and complications caused by the physician most likely cause a fever after the first week of surgery.

143. C: Lopressor is a beta-blocker which lowers blood pressure and heart rate. This can cause a variety of side effects such as dizziness and fatigue. Flushing can be seen with a number of medications such as niacin. Angioedema is commonly seen with ACE inhibitors. Patients may develop bruises easily if they are taking blood thinners or anti-platelet medications.

144. C: The patient's oxygenation status is normal. Although oxygenation status should always be monitored in a patient with sickle cell crisis, it is not an immediate concern at this time. The patient's blood pressure is low and IV fluids should be given. A complete blood count should also be checked to make sure that the patient isn't anemic. Pain and nausea should be addressed after the blood pressure is stabilized.

145. A: The nurse should remove the dressing and check the incision to make sure an infection is not present. After making sure that the incision looks normal, the nurse should inform the nurse manager of the incident and of the prior nurse's false documentation. The nurse should never falsely document anything; it is illegal, inappropriate, and it increases the risk of a negative outcome for the patient.

146. D: Cold temperatures can precipitate a sickle cell crisis, so cooling blankets should be avoided. If a patient has a fever, NSAIDs should be given. Sickle cell crises increase the risk for pulmonary embolus, stroke, and heart attack, so supplemental oxygen should always be given. Sickle cell crises are incredibly painful, so pain medications should be given. IV fluids help increase blood pressure and help protect the kidneys from damage.

147. B. All of the laboratory values are within normal limits except for the BUN, which is elevated to 26 from a normal of 7 to 17 mg/dL (reference values may vary somewhat). While this is outside the normal range, it is usually evaluated with creatinine to determine if there is kidney damage, and the creatinine level is normal. BUN values may be elevated by dehydration and some commonly-used drugs, such as acetaminophen and ibuprofen.

148. C: A common side effect of niacin is flushing. Niacin is used to raise a patient's high density lipoprotein (HDL) or their "good cholesterol." A patient should be started on the lowest dose possible to prevent adverse side effects. If flushing occurs, the drug does not necessarily have to be discontinued if the patient tolerates the side effect.

149. D: A mnemonic for remembering the common causes of post-operative fever is the five Ws: **w**ind (atelectasis, aspiration, pneumonia), **w**ater (urinary tract infection), **w**alking (deep vein thrombus), **w**ound (wound infection), **w**hat the physician caused (drug fever, line infection). Wind is most likely to cause a fever POD 1–2, water is most likely to cause a fever POD 3–5, walking is the most likely to cause a fever POD 5–7, wound is the most likely cause POD 5–9, and complications caused by the physician most likely cause a fever after the first week of surgery.

150. A: An aneurysm is the abnormal ballooning of the vessel wall due to weakness in the vasculature. Cigarette smoking is one of the primary causes of aneurysms, although they may also be caused by genetic disposition, increasing age (greater than 40 years old), and by certain diseases. The aneurysm was found in a young patient with no risk factors, so the immediate family members should be screened as soon as possible as a preventative measure. If anyone is found to have a cerebral aneurysm he/she can be monitored as an outpatient to make sure the aneurysm doesn't get bigger. Ruptured aneurysms may result in seizure, neurological compromise, and death.